River of Time

River of Time

My Descent into Depression
and How I Emerged With Hope

NAOMI JUDD

WITH MARCIA WILKIE

CENTER
STREET®

NEW YORK   BOSTON   NASHVILLE

Center Street
Hachette Book Group
1290 Avenue of the Americas, New York, NY 10104
centerstreet.com
twitter.com/centerstreet

First Edition: December 2016

Center Street is a division of Hachette Book Group, Inc. The Center Street name and logo are trademarks of Hachette Book Group, Inc.

The publisher is not responsible for websites (or their content) that are not owned by the publisher.

The Hachette Speakers Bureau provides a wide range of authors for speaking events. To find out more, go to www.HachetteSpeakersBureau.com or call (866) 376-6591.

Book design by Timothy Shaner/nightanddaydesign.biz

Library of Congress Cataloging-in-Publication Data has been applied for.

ISBNs: 978-1-4555-9574-7 (hardcover), 978-1-4555-9575-4 (ebook)

Printed in the United States of America

LSC-C

10   9   8   7   6   5   4   3   2   1

Even in the darkest days of my severe treatment resistant depression, I was never blinded to the compassion from my beloveds who continually reached down with loving hands and lifted me out of my harrowing nightmare of despair. Because of you, I can tell my story. I wrote it with the sincere hope of offering encouragement to the forty million Americans who suffer from depression and anxiety every minute of every day and night. I want them to know that I understand, and I'm here to help.

CONTENTS

CONTENTS

CONTENTS

FOREWORD

Many brilliant, amazing, talented individuals have suffered from depression, including Ludwig van Beethoven, Vincent van Gogh, Isaac Newton, Abraham Lincoln, Patty Duke, Jon Hamm, Billy Joel, Robin Williams, and Kirsten Dunst. Naomi is in good company. Of the ten professions most common among people who suffer depression, Naomi has devoted herself to two of the listed careers: entertainment, as a performer and writer, and the health care profession as an RN nurse.

When I first met Naomi, I was lecturing at a conference on complementary medicine, speaking on the connections between the brain, the mind, health, and intuition. I saw this woman, from a distance, who couldn't be overlooked. She had big red hair, full makeup, and a clothing style that very much set her apart from the "usual" crowd at these events. When my presentation was over, Naomi marched up to the podium and introduced herself. Later that day we had dinner. She invited me to visit her farm, and since that time, almost two decades ago, I've been making regular visits to Tennessee to stay with Naomi at "Peaceful Valley."

But Peaceful Valley hasn't always been so peaceful for Naomi, suffering a mind-body disorder like depression for more than three years, and for those of us who care about her. Yet, unquestionably, through the years when others of us—including me—have suffered our own health problems, Naomi has always been there. She is an unbeatable combination of intelligence, knowledge, personal experience, and compassion.

During the past years she has gone through unrelenting sadness, fatigue, panic, and insomnia. Still, Naomi pushes it aside to function—maybe even transcending the pain—to work, relate, love, and learn.

How is this possible? Let me try to explain.

Naomi's abundant talents in music, media, and communication, as well as her natural inclination toward stellar comprehension of medical knowledge and natural intuition, may bias her brain development in one direction, one that has generated her extraordinary life and career. The downside? Her immense sensitivity to environmental, social, and emotional nuance may, unfortunately, make her prone to depression. The great behavioral neurologist Dr. Norman Geschwind talked about the "pathology of superiority": When someone has an exceptional talent or skill in one part of his or her brain, another part of the brain may suffer. The most obvious examples of this are autistic savants, individuals who have an incredible capacity for attention to minutiae (left brain) but a developmental problem with social and emotional processing (right brain).

Perhaps you're thinking, Dr. Mona Lisa, use plain English, please. What are you saying? Well, the actual brain science can be simplified to a representative quote from my aunt Evie, a woman with a sixth-grade education who emigrated from Portugal. I never wanted to be like Aunt Evie, because she was uneducated, so I pursued my education to the highest achievements (PhD in neuroscience and an MD in psychiatry). She was simple folk. Though undereducated, Aunt Evie was very loving, compassionate, and intuitive, and possessed a valuable amount of common sense. Ironically, she described the connection between extreme talents and brain disorders in much the same way Dr. Geschwind did. Aunt Evie used to say, "I've never known a genius who didn't have a screw loose somewhere."

Aunt Evie's proclamation could describe us all. We all have some genius capacity in one area of our brain and a problem in another. Maybe your problem is depression, like Naomi's? Then one part of your healing may be to find out your unique genius that complements your uniquely sensitive, empathic, intuitive brain.

Naomi has an extremely fine-tuned brain. She was a registered nurse before beginning her music career, but definitely could have been a doctor. She devours medical literature, using a yellow highlighter and a slow, methodical method of taking notes, like a scanning electron microscope, taking in enormous amounts of scientific minutiae.

Naomi is actually ahead of her time. For more than a decade, she has told me about meeting with this noteworthy scientist or that scientist, this or that Nobel laureate, and so on. I used to wonder, how many of those scientific terms did Naomi really understand? Well, Naomi *really* understands those scientific terms from physics and medicine and more. One of the words that she used to toss around was *epigenetic*. I would think, Where did she get that word? When I was researching my latest book, I ran across the term *epigenetic* in a study on treating anxiety. Now in the latest scientific publications, news, and bestselling books we hear of the power of epigenetics and I am left to once again hand it to Naomi for being way ahead of her time.

There's another reason Naomi is highly qualified to write this book. Many people at Harvard, Stanford, the Mayo Clinic, the best universities and teaching hospitals, do research in labs or study patients in clinics, and they teach us about the brain and science. We may stand in awe of their minds and their genius. Is that what will help us understand suffering of the mind? Perhaps. In the last decade, psychiatry has made major inroads into medical treatment for major mental health afflictions. But when we're asking about these researchers' credentials—do they have an MD? a PhD? are they board-certified?—we may forget yet a final and oh so very important credential: Have they experienced the illness they treat?

Naomi has this credential. She has experienced severe depression and made major inroads into getting it treated. Yes, she has won many music industry awards and has created timeless music with her daughter Wynonna. Yes, as a nurse, she spent years studying the anatomy and physiology of the body. But one of Naomi's biggest credentials is that she has in fact suffered from depression, one of the most common and most significant disorders in humanity. I've watched her struggle with this illness, the ups and the downs and the sideways. I've seen medicines begin to work, then stop working. And through it all, I've seen Naomi's indomitable spirit.

I remember when I was first in medical school, I wanted to be a surgeon. It seemed that surgery could be so straightforward. You simply cut out what was wrong and stitched it up, or put some rods in. The first rotation that I went through was psychiatry, and I thought, Oh, this is the last thing I'd ever want to go into! But then my own spine fell apart, and suddenly I was the one who needed the rods put in. And as I figured out what further training I would need to get for a medical license, ultimately I ended up going into psychiatry simply because it was a branch of medicine in which I could sit down! Having since earned a PhD in neuroanatomy and behavioral neuroscience, I now ultimately have my practice in neuropsychiatry. I'm specifically poised to take a multifaceted view of all the treatments and the medicines prescribed to Naomi.

Of all the fields of medicine, psychiatry may be the most difficult, because it is in its infancy. Psychiatry is now where neurology was two decades ago. Whether it's the grossly unfair stigma or the lack of scans or blood tests to validate diagnoses, many people with depression, anxiety, moodiness, irritability, and so on suffer in silence or hide, for fear that people will think they're "touched." Well, I've been touched by watching Naomi valiantly struggle, and I'm touched that in writing this book she allows all of us, through her vulnerability, to see how she continues to fight this terrible disease of the brain.

Why do I say "continues"? It goes back to where I started this foreword.

Depression may be part and parcel of the "pathology of superiority." It may be the downside of the type of brain, the genius brain, that gives us the sensitivity and compassion we need for careers in entertainment and health care. In this, Naomi is perfectly poised to give you this book, whether it's through her knowledge of healing as a nurse, her sense of how to touch us with music and art, or the compassion she's developed for all of us who have suffered from one baffling ailment to another. Depression may be part and parcel of Naomi's genius.

You too may have your own ups and downs. You may use medicines, supplements, psychotherapies, prayer, and so on to try to heal your depression. Let Naomi's intelligence, knowledge, compassion, and personal experience give you hope that you *can* heal, and find your own genius, and have your own exceptional life.

—MONA LISA SCHULZ, MD, PHD
Author, *Heal Your Mind: Your Prescription for Wholeness Through Medicine, Affirmations, and Intuition* (Hay House, 2016)

River of Time

AUTHOR'S NOTE

Memory is often a subjective and imperfect recorder of details. My book is a stark look at my experiences of severe depression and anxiety and the treatments I underwent for both. I have brought forth the best of my recollections, though I am aware that my own memory is informed by the subject matter itself. It's rare for each of us to recall conversations exactly word for word. The ones that appear in the book have been paraphrased and convey my feelings and experience of them. We each have our own perceptions and realities. This is mine.

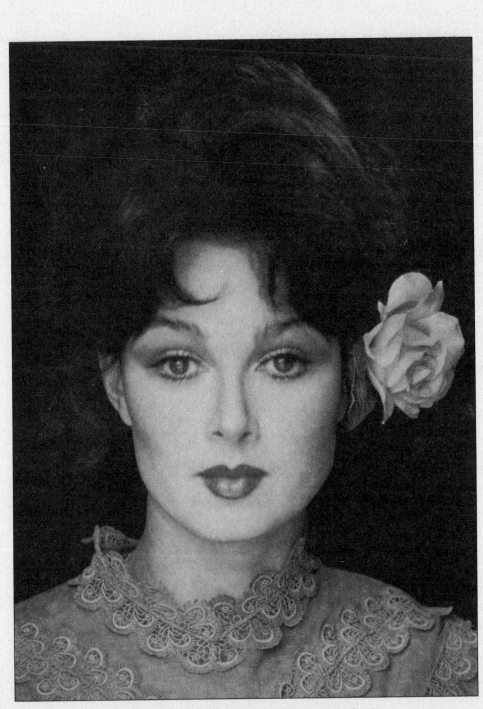

At twenty-two I was beaten and raped by an ex-con on heroin.
He passed out, which allowed me to escape with my life.

INTRODUCTION

I t's impossible to survive a 155-foot fall from a bridge over an asphalt highway. In 2013, I reached the conclusion that the only direction left for my worthless life was down. I was convinced that a sudden fall from a high bridge was better than the slow-motion emotional decline I was enduring day by day. I was drifting, alone in a murky ocean of guilt, anger, confusion, and unrelenting sorrow. I had done everything I could to climb out of it by following each psychiatrist's directions and giving any and all promising prescriptive cures a try. Nothing proved to be a lifeline I could grab. Nothing changed the reality that my once full and colorful life now looked empty and gray. I had tried "pulling myself up by the bootstraps," in true Judd style, for many months. But now I could no longer even stand up under the boulder-like weight of my severe treatment-resistant depression and terrifying panic attacks.

One bitterly cold and dreary morning the urgent thought came to me that if I couldn't get myself out of this despair, I should end my misery quickly. Death would be instantaneous relief. I would no longer be an emotional burden to my family and friends. I was in such a state of serious brain fog that I wasn't able to consider the effect my suicide would have on my fans. I imagined that the impact of my body hitting the highway would leave me unrecognizable. It would be a logical end, because I no longer recognized myself.

The world knows me as the Mom half of the Judds singing duo. My daughter Wynonna and I were the most documented and commercially successful duo act in the history of country music during the 1980s and some of the 1990s. The public saw me in concert, singing and dancing at world-famous venues from Carnegie Hall to the London Palladium, the Houston Astrodome to Madison Square Garden. We performed for the millions of people who watched Super Bowl XXVIII, as the 72,000 football fans filling the Georgia Dome sang along to the popular ballad I had written, "Love Can Build a Bridge." The Judds' singles were number one hits, fourteen topped the Hot Country Songs chart, and our albums went platinum, selling more than 20 million worldwide. We were undefeated at every awards show, with eight Country Music Association awards. The Judds won six Grammys and I won my own, as writer of the "Best Country Song."

Then, just when we were cresting the top of the show business world, in 1990, doctors told me that I had only three years to live. I had been diagnosed with hepatitis C, which I had unknowingly contracted while working as a nurse, before the Judds took off. The virus usually takes several years to produce severe symptoms.

Born an optimist, I chose to not accept the fate with which the doctors had sealed my future. I was offended by their "curse" of a rapid decline. I angrily rebelled as if a medical hex had been placed on me. As an RN I've witnessed what can happen when a doctor gives a patient a grim prognosis. All too often the diagnosis determines the outcome of the disease. Our beliefs become our biology.

I had been on my own since the age of seventeen. I learned very early in life that when anything went wrong, I was the one who had to take charge and figure out what I needed to do to survive. Now I was very sick, but I faced hepatitis C with my fists up. There was no known cure at that time, so all I could do was fight to survive.

I spent the next couple of decades learning about the human brain and the state of neuroscience, delving into the findings of brilliant researchers who were making breakthroughs on the mind, body, and spirit connection. I applied to my own life everything I was learning about how our personal beliefs affect our body, mind, and spirit. I met with many of these scholars and doctors, even Nobel Prize–winning geniuses in medicine like Dr. Francis Collins, who decoded the human genome and is now the director of the National Institutes of Health, and consider many of them to be my friends. Books on the most cutting-edge discoveries in science and health would predictably be found stacked on the night table beside my bed.

I have always been intrigued by health care and thought it would be my lifelong career when I was a single mother with two young daughters. My plan was to work full-time as a nurse and find a way to enroll in medical school at the University of Louisville, in my home state of Kentucky. I wanted to work with underserved people in the Appalachian region. My plan was set aside, unexpectedly, when Wynonna and I began singing in public and were encouraged to perform more often. After every appearance audience members would inquire why we weren't already living in Nashville. Singing was and is the only career Wynonna ever desired. Performing is what she does brilliantly. As her mom, I knew we had to move to Nashville, to give Wynonna the best chance at a career in music. I believed her destiny was already stamped on her forehead. Yet my own interest in holistic medicine never waned.

By 1995 doctors proclaimed me completely free of the hepatitis C virus. I felt radiantly healthy again and buoyantly happy. I wrote a book about my miraculous recovery and became a sought-after speaker on many topics. I had gained a comprehensive understanding of the body-mind-spirit connection and was asked by professional medical and social service organizations to be a keynote speaker at their national gatherings. I was honored to pass along any information that could possibly help someone else. My point of view was that there could always be healing, even if there isn't always a cure. At the same time, I had a national talk radio show on Sirius XM, a Sunday morning talk show for Hallmark Channel taped in New York, and was cast in a number of made-for-TV movies. I was thrilled to be busy every day of the week.

Still, the fans demanded a reunion of the Judds. At their request, Wynonna and I paired up for a North American tour in 2000, called "The Power to Change" tour. The response was overwhelming and the enthusiasm of the sold-out crowds was electrifying.

Then, in 2010, we came together for another widely antici-pated tour. The Oprah Winfrey Network (OWN) heard about our plans and requested the opportunity to film our "Encore" tour, both behind the scenes and onstage. The resulting footage would be a reality show for the launch of the inaugural season of Oprah's new network.

My life was filled with interesting people, different scenery, new things to learn, and exhilarating events. I had plenty of reasons to jump out of bed every morning. Never did I expect that only months after the Encore tour ended I would feel I had every reason to jump off a bridge to end my tortured existence.

How could that be possible? I've asked myself that question countless times. I had always been an eternal optimist. I was thought of as the caring, wise one with the sympathetic ear, whom everyone else came to for encouragement and answers. Who had time to be depressed? But depression had time for me, stole time from me.

This book is the story of two and a half years of my life, during which I went through the hell of mental illness. It isn't just about a victorious recovery, but about a wary and humble gratitude for persevering through thirty terrifying months and regaining hope and a purpose for living once more. It's the account of hitting rock bottom and rising again to be thankful for taking my next breath, for the gift of a clear thought, for wresting from a nightmare a way to find joy in each day.

You might question how someone in my situation, with my financial and educational resources, could have languished for two and a half years without a resolution to my depression and anxiety. Before 2011, I would have asked the same question.

Isn't America a medically and technically advanced country, where almost everything can be treated? This may be true for many of our physical illnesses, but in the United States, treatment for mental illness lags far behind the advancements made in other countries. According to Dr. Allen Frances, professor emeritus and former chairman of the department of psychiatry and behavioral sciences at Duke University, "For people with severe mental illness, there has never been a time and a place worse than now in the United States." (*New York Times*, October 20, 2015.)

I learned the hard way that mental health issues cover a wide scope of disorders and can be hard to diagnose. No one can see or easily pinpoint the problem because it's all in the mind. Unlike a broken arm, there's nothing to detect in an X-ray. There are 100 billion neurons in the human brain. Christof Koch, the world-renowned neuroscientist who is the chief scientific officer at the renowned Allen Institute in Seattle, has described the brain as "the most complex object in the universe."

Adding to the difficulty, many types of anxiety and depression have been identified. Dr. Daniel Amen, a double-board-certified psychiatrist and neuroscientist, names seven:

1. Pure anxiety
2. Pure depression
3. Mixed anxiety and depression: This is the case for 75 percent of people who suffer.
4. Overfocused anxiety and depression: when you get stuck on negative thoughts or behavior
5. Unfocused anxiety and depression: low energy, brain fog, lack of attention span
6. Cyclic anxiety and depression: mild to serious mood swings
7. Temporal lobe anxiety and depression: result of a head injury or seizures

Psychiatrists now realize that depression and anxiety are more commonly found together than separately. Only about one-third of sufferers are treated for both.

In my case, I was unaware that I had post-traumatic stress disorder from pathological situations and issues passed down through generations along with the traumatic events of my own life. I felt humiliated and emotionally weak and I deluded myself that I could pull out of it alone because I've always been such a strong-willed woman. I denied the problem and it lingered until it became unbearable. Finally, others forced me to get help. Unfortunately, I wasn't in a good place, emotionally or mentally, to choose the best treatment for myself.

The stigma around mental illness comes with the dangerous and erroneous message that we are weak in character and that we should be able to "snap out of it." Wrong! It's a brain disease. Depression and panic attacks are not signs of weakness. The chemical imbalance in the brain is very real and it takes both understanding and courage to live with it until a trained psychiatrist can figure out a course of treatment. The worst thing you can say to a depressed patient is "Just snap out of it!"

Because I survived, I feel a responsibility to share what brought me hope and what's kept me alive. What carried me toward recovery was the relatively recent discovery by geneticists like Dr. Francis Collins and neuroscientists that only one-third of your genes are actually inherited from your family of origin. The good news is that you can alter about two-thirds of your genes by making good choices, even if you were born into a long line of pathological, depressed, mentally ill, and even suicidal family members, like I was.

I certainly wasn't alone in my despair. Twenty million people in the United States suffer from one of the forms of depression (350 million worldwide), and two-thirds of us wait too long to seek help. Forty million of us have legitimate anxiety disorders that can shatter our peace of mind. Suicides outnumber homicides every single year. In June 2013, the Centers for Disease Control and Prevention showed that suicides among middle-aged people have gone up nearly 50 percent since 1999. Roughly twenty of our brave veterans commit suicide every day. For women over age sixty, the rate rose by 60 percent. With the divorce rate between 40 and 50 percent, nearly nine million people being displaced by downsizing and layoffs (especially for those over age fifty), and the social isolation created by our transient, fractured society, there are millions of people who feel "dumped." Baby boomers, who number over 76 million, are the largest demographic in the United States and also the most depressed age group. Antidepressants are the third most common medication taken by Americans, according to the National Health and Nutrition Examination Survey, including 23 percent of women over age forty.

At the same time, our life expectancy in the United States has risen to an all-time high. What are we to do with the last twenty or thirty years of our lives? Who can serve as examples of living with purpose and happiness, if so few have ever lived as long as many of us likely will? When the children are grown and gone, the source of your livelihood has come to an end, and the busyness of a daily full schedule has diminished, what is left to give you a sense of purpose?

I wasn't prepared for this new chapter in my life. It opened the gateway to severe loneliness, depression, and anxiety. I had never identified or processed the hidden trauma of my past, the pathology of my family of origin, and it moved into my open calendar to demand my full attention every agonizing day and night.

As you will read in this book, I have had to excavate long-buried feelings about my family ties. Because I grew up in a household where the mottos were "That's just the way it is" and "Don't talk about it," anger and resentment had a lifelong grip on me that I wasn't fully able to accept until I was willing to open up and get treatment for my depression and anxiety.

I was stunned by how many of my adult reactions were in response to my early programming by my parents and older relatives. As a typical firstborn child, trying to satisfy my relatives' expectations and create happiness for them became my daily and ultimately my lifetime goal. I set unreasonable benchmarks of perfection for myself. Any dip below those standards created another layer of unresolved guilt.

I know that our perceptions are always subjective and that what is true for one may not be at all true for another. Each of us has a perception of how another person treats us. That person has their perception of us, as well. The two realities are rarely the same. Although my siblings were born of the same parents and raised in the same household, we have very different perceptions of reality and, as a result, have become very different adults.

However, to help myself heal I had to accept that my feelings were true for me. I had always pushed my negative feelings far down in my psyche and labeled them as odd or self-indulgent because I was told, as a child, that they were. I know there are reasons each of us becomes who we are and why we do what we do. By the time a child is three years old her self-image is formed.

My own daughters have each spoken publicly and written about how their childhood experiences and growing up with me as their mother had both a positive and a negative effect on the adults they have become. The good memories they have of the three of us make me smile. For any sad or angry memory they have, I can truthfully declare, "If I had known better, I would have done better." I think that is true of most people, but not all. For example, people with a narcissistic personality disorder or borderline personality disorder may know better, but are often too self-absorbed to be able to do better.

The unarguable fact is that we are responsible for our actions and our reactions, too. You can be inactive, reactive, or proactive. As an adult, understanding this helped me to uncover and directly face what I experienced as a child. There were so many buried feelings that I couldn't develop healthy emotions. It's not my intention to incriminate my relatives. What I want is to identify, accept, and heal my own long-held pain from these unprocessed experiences. For me, it's a matter of life and death.

Long before recorded history, storytelling was the way one generation passed along news, gossip, insight, and humor. Often the stories carried hard-earned wisdom, meant to spare the next generation the heartache the elders had been through. The stories also connect us to the range of human experience.

I am giving you my unvarnished story, to encourage you to look at every past and current aspect of who you are today, whether you suffer depression or simply want to lead a more fulfilling life. I hope my story will encourage you to begin your own voyage of self-discovery leading to wholeness of body, mind and spirit.

Change is the true nature of this world. Change will happen for all of us. We can find our way out of self-punishment, anger, and depression. My case is extreme, so if I can make lifesaving changes, I know you can, too.

Chapter 1
Shhh...Don't Tell a Soul

t's not a bad dream or even a horror movie nightmare, though it has become the most harrowing aspect of what is now my constant personal torment.

It's three in the morning and I go from a deep sleep to standing bolt upright on my bed, the covers draped around my feet like the Statue of Liberty, but I am not free. I am imprisoned in my body; my mind has taken me hostage in ways that are unbelievably terrifying. I reach up to my throat, expecting to find a pair of hands belonging to an intruder who is out to kill me with a grip that is slowly closing down on my windpipe. I am hyperventilating. My heart is beating so rapidly that my eardrums are throbbing. I am in danger, but I don't know the reason why. My vision blurs. The room spins. My face, neck, chest, and palms are covered with sweat.

My terror, which seems to send lightning bolts of energy through our perfectly quiet bedroom, awakens my husband abruptly. My dog Bijou, who has been snuggled next to me, jumps from the bed yelping wildly, which brings the other two dogs, Maudie and Lulu, racing into the room. All three dogs are in protective mode, looking for a dangerous intruder. They sniff at the doors and scamper down the hallways, fur on their backs raised, ready to attack.

The intruder is here in the panic, which is rising up with a vicious force inside me, breaking through six decades of suppression. The intruder has had enough of living in a stifled memory far below

11

my optimistic consciousness and is here to follow through with what he started. He's here for the lonely toddler who never trusted that she could tell anyone her truth, not even her mother. He has come for Naomi Ellen Judd, the sweet Appalachian child, and he's not going away this time, no matter how hard I've tried to forget about what happened long before my first day of kindergarten.

I am no longer Naomi Judd, the mother of two daughters, the mom half of the Judds, the most documented act and successful singing duo in the history of country music. I haven't yet won a Grammy or Country Music Association award or had platinum albums and number one singles. I haven't had sold out concerts at the London Palladium, Madison Square Garden, or the Houston Astrodome. I'm no longer married to my life partner and true love of thirty-seven years, gospel singer and former backup singer for Elvis Presley, Larry Strickland. I'm not in the warm, comfortable bed we share in our beautiful home in the lush countryside of Franklin, Tennessee.

No, I have been emotionally transported back, to my very first memory, as a toddler, in my dreary, gray, and somber hometown of Ashland, Kentucky.

The eruptive memory of this unwelcome life-altering experience has overtaken my mind, in the much the same way the Ohio River can rise and overflow into Ashland with muddy swirling water whenever there is a significant storm. Positioned on the border of West Virginia and Ohio, Ashland often suffers severe weather that lingers, brought to a standstill between the Appalachian Mountains. During my childhood, the sun also had to compete with the layer of fine black particles that always settled to the ground after hanging in the damp air.

Three major industrial plants based their production in Ashland, taking advantage of the fierce Ohio River. The majority of

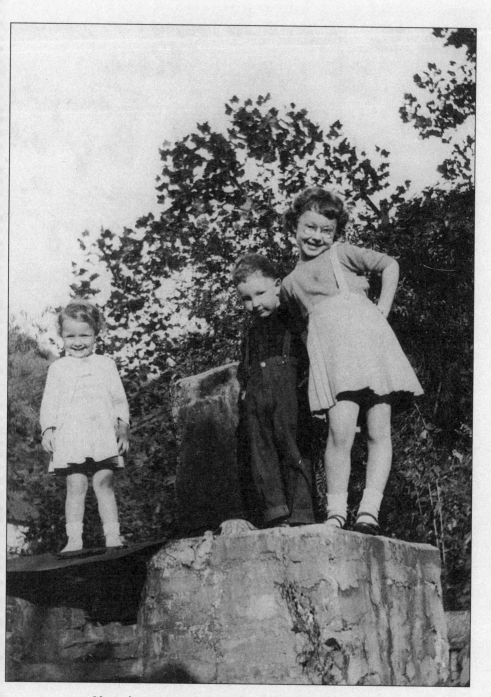

I learned at a young age to be a polite child with a sweet disposition,
despite the dark secret that was crushing my sense of safety.

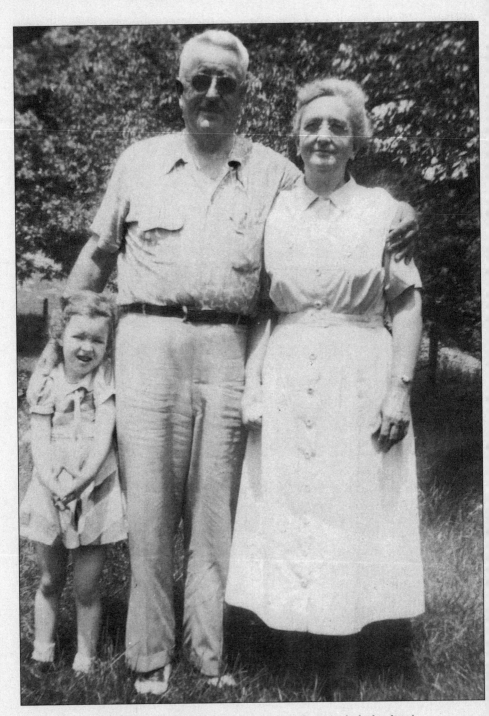

Grandmommy Judd forced me to stand next to the man who had molested me months before this photo. I am, obviously, terrified of Uncle Charlie.

Ashland men worked at one of these plants, many spending their workdays filling large ovens with tons of coal, baking it into the fuel called coke. As a result, the community had to live with heavy pollutants and a constant noxious odor. A layer of black soot, which coated our windowsills and most likely our lungs, was ever-present. Even sitting on a park bench was out of the question, unless you took the time to wipe off the grime.

In the 1950s, doctors were still unaware of the causes of lung cancer and other diseases toxins create in the body. Living with this pollution was just the way things were. For me, my hometown was not only a place of darkened skies and a stagnant stench; it was also a sealed vault of fetid family secrets.

On this winter night in Franklin, Tennessee, decades after I left Ashland, my subconscious has figured out the combination to unlock the vault and drag the heavy door open. The secrets have escaped to destroy my sleep. They play across my mind's eye like a virtual reality video game. It feels so real that I could reach out and touch it. My mind had been proficient at keeping the shameful secrets suppressed, so why are they emerging now as a nocturnal panic attack, surfacing from my slumbering subconscious as if past events were happening in my own bedroom? I can hear the whisper, "Shhh…don't tell a soul."

I am three and a half years old and running a high fever. My small toddler body is aflame with fire-red chicken pox. My pregnant mother has deposited me with her Judd in-laws to prevent me from infecting my two-year-old brother, Brian, at home. She can't stand her in-laws or anyone on Daddy's side of the family, something I am well aware of. However, they live only two blocks away and are the only nearby solution to her problem, me. I have been sent to stay with Grandmommy Judd in my flannel nightgown, which is torture against my feverish, itchy skin. Grandmommy sternly warns me to not scratch as she points the way to the tall feather bed in the small attic room at the end of squeaky, wood-planked hallway, and instructs me to stay in it. I have to figure out a way to climb in, by myself, though the mattress top is at my eye level.

I grab the iron bedpost and dig my toes into the edge of the frame until I boost myself high enough to get my knees on top of the mattress. I crawl to the center and under the covers. I rest my head on a fat feather pillow and listen to the domestic sounds coming from the house. I can tell that my four eccentric adult aunts, all of whom still live with Grandmommy and Granddaddy, are bustling about doing their chores. I feel like my face is burning, yet I'm shivering at the same time. I'm tempted to scratch the red bumps that have banished me to my grandmother's bed, alone and sick, but I won't. I'm already an exceptionally well-behaved child, doing whatever she's told, searching for a sign of approval.

While everyone is wrapped up in housework, I am feeling abandoned and restless with fever. Then, I hear the squeak of the floorboards in the hallway. I have a trace of hope that it's Mother, coming back to get me. I want her to comfort me, to lift me up in her arms, and take me home. But I know that is highly unlikely. She hasn't held me on her lap since the day I learned to walk. She never reads me bedtime stories or tucks me in. Everything my mother does for me is done with practicality. The only time she touches me is to run a brush through my wavy hair in the morning, tugging at the tangles, or to yank up the zipper of my jacket before she shoos me outside.

I know it's not Mother coming to see me. Instead, I start to imagine that the person coming down the hallway will be Daddy. He's heard that I'm sick and has come to take me home. I want the footsteps to be Daddy's work boots. I always felt my Daddy loved me. But I know he is working at his small gas station and it would be too much for him to close his business, our livelihood, to look in on a lonely, sick little girl.

The door slowly creaks open. It's a male figure looming in the hallway. I know instantly that it's not Daddy. I turn over on my side, as close to the wall as possible, and scrunch my knees up toward my chest. I am hoping this old man who is peering in at me will go away. I dread the sound of the door being closed, because I know the man is now inside the room. I'm a captive. I squeeze my eyes shut, praying that if I pretend to be asleep, he will leave. I can hear the sound of a belt buckle coming loose, then a zipper. His stale breath comes out in short, noisy puffs. I have no reference point for what is about to happen to me, but my infantile innate senses tell me that the survival of my soul is at stake.

I pull the sheets up around my neck and press my tiny body as close to the wall as possible. I sense that the other side of the sheets and blanket are being lifted. The mattress sinks down and the bedsprings make an off-key sound like an out-of-tune Autoharp as the intruder climbs into bed beside me. I can smell hair tonic, cigarettes, and musty body odor. I turn to see that it's Uncle Charlie, my Grandma Judd's brother. He places his finger to his mouth and says, "Shhh."

He reaches under the sheet and grabs the calf of my leg and drags me across the mattress toward his body. I can feel the chicken pox on my back rupturing open from being yanked across the stiff cotton sheets. As I am pulled closer I can see that his pants are undone and his privates are exposed. Of course, I've never seen adult male genitals before. His breathing is even heavier, which scares me so much I hold my own breath. He has an odd and creepy grin in the face of my terror. He uses his dirty rough hands to push my nightgown up to my underarms and then grabs at my waist to pull me toward him. In that very moment, at age three and a half, I understand that no one is going to save me from Uncle Charlie. I have to save myself.

I jerk my arms out from under the sheet and grab the flesh of his face in my hands. I dig my fingernails into the soft baggy skin under his eyes. Then I manage to bring a foot up and jab it into his throat, right at his Adam's apple. Uncle Charlie coughs in surprise and lets go of me. I scramble to sit up on the bed and then scoot back away from him until I awkwardly tumble off the end of the mattress and drop with a loud thump to the floor.

I'm scared witless that Uncle Charlie will catch up to me at the door, but he doesn't. He is probably equally afraid that someone has heard the thump of my fall and will open the door to find him exposed. His face is now red-streaked from my scratch marks. I yank at the doorknob that I can barely turn, open it, and run along the hallway and down the stairs to the back porch and then out into the cool dusk. Two of my aunts, Evelyn and Ramona, are there shaking out rugs against the back fence. They don't see the look of pure fear on my face. It seems that doing mundane chores is far more import-ant than a terror-stricken little girl.

Uncle Charlie isn't looking for me anymore. He has his floppy hat that he always wears pulled low over his face and he waves good-bye to my aunts from the sidewalk and leaves quickly.

I go back inside and peer up at the wrinkled and tired face of my Grandmommy Judd, who is standing at the kitchen sink. She has a bandana tied around her forehead, the sign that she's suffering another migraine headache. The steam is rising from the hot water in the dishpan and streaming down the window over the sink like long tears on a sad face. What will happen if I tell her? I don't know what words to use. I have no way to comprehend what Uncle Charlie was trying to do to me. I only knew it was wrong.

Grandmommy Judd looks down at me after I tug on the hem of her dress gently. I search her face, longing for her to see my terror and make me feel safe somehow. I hope she will ask me, "What's wrong, sweetheart?" when she sees how frightened I am. I don't find comfort in her eyes, only frustration with being bothered. Grandmommy Judd frowns, raises her eyebrows in a disapproving way, wipes her hands on her apron, and points me back upstairs. I can't go in that room, again. I stand against the refrigerator, frozen in fear.

Should I run the two blocks barefoot to our home, crossing a busy street by myself, and tell Mother? I already know that her reaction will be one of anger. She never wants to have to interact with the Judds about any issue.

Anytime I expressed emotions, whether they were joyful, fearful, or full of hope, Mother would become annoyed. I knew she would be mad at me for causing trouble. Even at age three and a half, I understood that my mother didn't seem interested in whatever happened to me. The one person on earth who was supposed to love and watch out for me didn't. My hope of being protected was crushed.

Tiny Naomi Ellen Judd had no one to tell. No one cared. I fully realized that I was on my own. Live or die, make or break, it all rested on my will. I wasn't going to die or break. Somehow, I would live. At this early age I possessed the character trait of persistence: There would be nothing I wouldn't try to live down, rise above, or overcome. For my very young self, it meant that the experience of being sexually assaulted couldn't be allowed to stick in my memory if I were to survive intact.

I submerged this crushing secret to the very bottom of my subconscious. How many more Uncle Charlies might be lurking out there? I would come to find out there were more, one even worse.

Yet, here I was, six decades later, at a time in my life when I should be enjoying the bounty of my successes and my unimaginably exciting career, panicked, in the middle of the night. Living a past trauma as if it all were happening again.

Larry pulls at my hand to sit down on the edge of the bed so he can rub my back, but I can't stay still. If I do I'm certain my heart will overload. I can't breathe well enough to tell him that I am coming apart. Am I losing my mind? The dogs whine and sniff at my feet as I walk to the bedroom door. I can barely feel my limbs, but I move into the hallway. I walk from room to room, never stopping. The dogs follow me, until they realize that I'm not going to settle down. They give up on me an hour later and jump back up on the bed with Larry for the rest of the night. I am too afraid to go to sleep. I don't want to find myself back in the memory of that feather bed. I keep moving.

When the morning light starts coming through the windows, I am exhausted. I finally sit at the kitchen table as Larry comes down the stairs. I can tell he is extremely worried, but he tries his best to make it seem like any other normal day. He puts on a pot of coffee and then whistles to the dogs to go out. Larry takes out his Bible to read a chapter or two in the same way he does every single morning. It fortifies him. He asks me if I'd like to pray about whatever kept me up the whole night before. I can't answer him. My mind feels too messed up to plug into anything about God, but I don't know how to admit that to a man whose faith has never wavered. I manage to mumble, "Later." Larry pulls on his jacket to go out to the barn to feed the cats and horses. As soon as he opens the back door, frigid, damp air rushes in. It's another gray and dreary day; one seems to follow another. I drag myself over to the couch near our big kitchen table and collapse under a throw blanket, pulling it up to my chin. I wonder what all of this stress is doing to my health.

While recovering from hepatitis C fifteen years ago, I learned that unbridled stress can wreak havoc on every system of your body, including the immune system, and precipitate many types of illnesses. According to facts quoted by Dr. Andrew Weil, physician and bestselling author, 90 percent of all visits to primary care physicians are due to stress-related illness. Andy is responsible for sterling research on mind-body-spirit medicine and has personally taught me so much. I had become quite expert at controlling what my mind would say to my body. I had to. The doctors had told me I would die in three years from hepatitis C. I rejected that message and my liver responded in a positive way. But this time there was no doctor giving me bad news.

My panic attacks are a manifestation of a past crisis hidden in my subconscious. The current message arising from my sleep-starved mind is, "It's hopelessly over for you, Naomi Ellen Judd. Underneath your upbeat public personality is a ravaged and fragmented young girl whom you've spent decades trying to forget."

There is someone I wish I could call, someone with whom I once shared everything, who has been with me through most of my trials and all of my successes. She has witnessed me overcoming many challenges in the past. I want this person to come over and just be with me today. I'm in such emotional danger I would love for her to comfort me and encourage me to believe that I will be fine no matter what. I know better. My wishes are as futile as those of the three-year-old Naomi Ellen Judd, hoping Mother would come to comfort her and rescue her from being molested and tell her she can beat hep C. It's not going to happen now because it has never happened in the past. I know she won't be calling me. We have barely spoken to each other in almost two years.

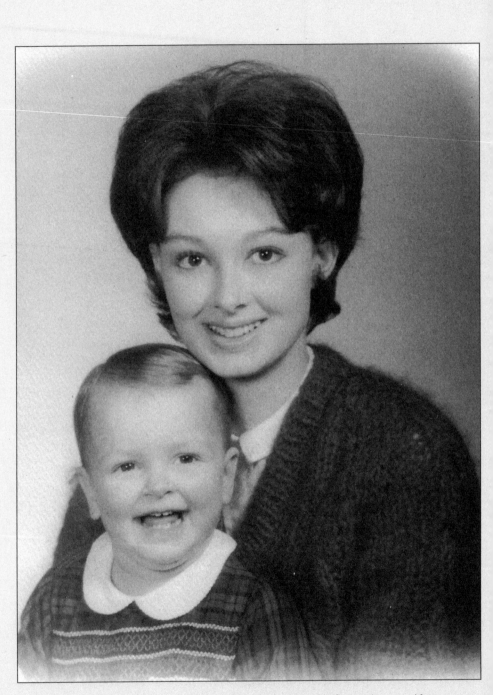

*I was a full-time nineteen-year-old mother, getting by in my in-laws attic room with my
baby, while my absent husband was living the fun student life in a college dorm.*

Chapter 2
Leaving Home

She left an old photograph of the two of us in my mailbox. It's a snapshot of me, age eighteen, in 1964, holding her as a newborn. I'm sitting on a couch in my in-laws' living room. My hair is teased a foot high and I am wearing one of the three dresses I owned. My husband, Michael, isn't in the picture because he was away at college and appeared to be footloose and fancy free while fraternizing with other students, leading a double life. I had been left behind to live in his parents' home, up in a small attic room with slanted ceilings. My back ached from crouching over so much, holding a baby in my arms. I could only stand up straight in the exact center of the room.

In 1960 (an innocent time in our country) I was a naïve fifteen-year-old girl who was being courted by Michael Ciminella, a nice-looking older boy, who seemed smitten with me. I was flattered. He was an only child whose parents belonged to the country club, lived in a beautiful home with a full china cabinet, and had hired a woman to clean their house once a week. Michael had everything I craved, most of all parents who adored him and would have done anything to make him happy. I couldn't even imagine what that would be like.

He attended an elite military school out of state. When Michael was home, he still wore his uniform and cap all the time, turning the heads of many girls as he cruised the streets of Ashland in a brand-new baby blue Chrysler Imperial. I felt like a princess riding around our small town in that expensive, piece-of-art car. My friends were impressed.

As a full year passed, and I had matured a bit more, I realized I had been blinded by the image of his privileged life and not by him. I didn't respect Michael, despite the fact that he was in constant pursuit of me and was determined I would be his. He was very used to getting his way. He asked me to marry him on our first date. I guess he was thinking that if Jerry Lee Lewis could marry a thirteen-year-old, then what was the problem with fifteen? I wasn't having it at fifteen or sixteen. It was a different story at seventeen, when marriage was my only solution.

In the photo that was left in my mailbox, I'm looking up at the camera with an anxious, yet compliant, smile, an eighteen-year-old who has been plunged into a responsibility that overwhelmed and frightened her. I saw myself as imprisoned and doomed to a life of housework, ironing, and washing diapers. The lonely, young, inexperienced mother in that photo could never have predicted her own future: that in twenty years this fragile infant and I would become a famous singing duo. I couldn't have foreseen that my firstborn girl would be blessed with a singing voice that would stir the souls of millions of people.

Yet now, at this traumatic and confusing point in my life, I seldom hear that beautiful familiar voice. I rarely see her, in person, even though she lives on a farm just over the hill, less than a mile away. This is the only way she feels safe communicating with me, a photo in the mailbox and an occasional text message.

I prop the yellowing photo in a prominent place on the hallway table and wonder why she chose this one to leave for me. Does she see the same thing in this photo that I see? Is she looking at the baby or the girl? Because that's what I was when I gave birth to her, a girl, a terrified teenager, in many ways as helpless as her baby. A year before this picture was taken, I had been going to sleepovers and football games with my high school girlfriends.

I had a deep and unbreakable love for my new daughter the second I laid eyes on her, but I still felt a deep inner conflict about coming to terms with the drastic life change I was experiencing. I had no idea what the future held for us. I only knew it was now the two of us against the world. With no one to talk to, I was left to painfully ruminate over the previous year, which had permanently altered the course of my life from the girlhood I knew only eleven months earlier. Once again, it was obvious that no one would be reaching out to me in sympathy or with advice. I was the one who had disappointed my family by getting pregnant, so I couldn't allow myself an ounce of self-pity.

Everything rapidly started to change in 1963, the year I was seventeen, in a confusing and scary way when my younger brother, Brian, became terminally ill. He had been hiding a growing tumor on his shoulder. It was obvious that it was serious when our family doctor sent him to a specialist in Ohio. Once he was diagnosed, my parents had a silent but united focus on getting Brian medical help. They spent many days away, driving back and forth to Columbus, to be at the hospital with my brother as he began treatments.

My parents would never discuss the situation with me, even when I pleaded to know what the doctors were telling them. They acted as if not talking about Brian's illness would make it go away, or at least somehow make it easier for all of us. I could have predicted that they would respond in this manner. I had resigned myself to the reality that "not talking about it" was the way my parents dealt with anything that was difficult to face. I'm not sure that Brian ever knew his own diagnosis or what was wrong with him. At a time when I ached for us to be a close family, to fall into each other's arms, shed many tears, and support each other through this nightmare, the exact opposite happened. We each went to our separate corners of denial. Mom would stay in the kitchen. Daddy would be at his gas station for twelve hours every day. Brian's red hair fell out and he would lie on the couch with a bucket nearby for his constant nausea.

My younger brother and sister didn't seem to comprehend what was going on at all. I tried to occupy myself with getting ready for my last year of high school, but it was a lonely endeavor, especially knowing that Brian wouldn't be going back to school with me. I felt powerless to help my good-humored, redheaded best buddy.

Desperate to emotionally connect with someone who would understand my fears, I took an opportunity that knocked on my door on the night of my greatest heartache. My parents were on a two-day trip to the hospital in Columbus with Brian. My little brother and sister were staying overnight with our neighbor, who volunteered to get them to school in the morning. For the very first time in my seventeen years, I was home alone. I had let Charlie Jordan, a good-looking high school football player, know that I was at my house and very sad about my brother's worsening health. I was hoping to distract myself from my worries by flirting with Charlie if he stopped by.

I was flattered when he showed up and was full of compliments about how attractive he thought I was. I wanted to believe his compliments and saw them as an opening to become his girlfriend. I was happy to be held in his arms. But, it turned into much more than that. I was caught up in his desire and beyond having reasonable judgment.

By the time he went home an hour later, he had taken my virginity and left me in far worse emotional shape than ever before. I felt depleted, full of shame, and robbed of my innocence. I spent a sleepless night, one of many, wondering why I let my first time happen that way: no true romance, no flowers, and no commitments. I had no choice but to go to school the next day, although I was terrified that my friends could see my shocking secret written all over my face.

As my brother's life was ending, I unknowingly began a new life inside me from that one sexual experience with Charlie, one night that was never to be repeated. Three months later, after figuring out a way to see a doctor secretly, I had to face the fact that I had become pregnant. I took my allowance from my piggy bank and called the one cab in town, since I hadn't learned to drive yet. It was November 25, 1963, the same day America buried President John F. Kennedy. The country reeled with the abrupt end of the hopes and dreams of a young leader. I was doing the same on a personal level. My hopes of being a carefree teenager, going to school dances, and dancing to the Beatles' "I Want to Hold Your Hand" had come to an abrupt end.

Not knowing what to do, I found Charlie Jordan after school one day and told him my dilemma. That was the last time I ever saw or spoke to him. He packed up and disappeared. I heard, by word of mouth, that he had moved to Pikeville and was working for the railroad.

My sense of security was completely shaken, because I knew I couldn't trust anyone to give me guidance. Mother was the one person I longed to go to, but there was no doubt in my mind that she would be too upset about Brian to worry about what this experience would mean for me or what should be done.

I had no loving adult to give me advice or guidance, so I kept my secret all to myself for the first four months. Finally, when I was almost five months along, Mom confronted me. Instead of uniting with me to figure out what would be best for my future and her upcoming grandchild's, she heartlessly kicked me out of the house during my fifth month of pregnancy. I had my hands on my growing belly as Mother flatly said, "You can't live here anymore. I can't have a crying baby in this house."

That night, as I struggled to accept Mother's unwavering decision, I went into my childhood bedroom, closed the door, lay across my bed, and wept for myself for the first time over this situation. I longed to have the chance to finish my senior year of high school with my classmates, read books, write papers, and do whatever other seventeen-year-olds were doing. I had only days to figure out where I could possibly go and how I would support myself and the new baby, since I didn't have a job or a place to live.

I had often heard the saying "Better the devil you know than the devil you don't know" and now felt that I had no choice but to accept Michael Ciminella's long-standing proposal to marry him. He knew his parents would be happy to have a daughter-in-law and a new grandchild, believing it was Michael's baby, on the way. With great sadness, I left behind my own fractured family, my bedroom with all of my dolls and collection of perfume bottles, my high school pals, and any fantasy of going to college at the University of Kentucky.

Living in the Ciminella's home, I went from having very little attention as a child to having more attention and opinionated direction than I could patiently handle. Even though obsessive-compulsive disorder was not recognized and listed in the *Diagnostic and Statistical Manual of Mental Disorders* until 1968, I'm dead certain that Mrs. Ciminella was the textbook definition. I felt like I was at the mercy of a meticulous home economics instructor. Every waking minute was filled with directions on the proper and correct way to do everything, from ironing a shirt to squeezing a toothpaste tube. I spent thirty minutes with her after each meal, as she repeated the "rules" of washing the dishes: glassware first, silverware next, then plates. I wanted to scream at her, grab my baby, and run into the woods.

The first day home from the hospital, Mrs. Ciminella insisted that we all wear surgical masks. I'm not kidding. She had sanitized the house from floor to ceiling. If I brought anything new into the house she sprayed it down with Lysol disinfectant. She was always checking to see if my hands were recently washed and if my finger-nails were short and spotlessly clean before I could touch my own baby. She would keep a thermometer on the floor to make sure it was warm enough when Wy was in her playpen. My new mother-in-law was always at my elbow, with instructions on how to care for my infant "the right way."

Anytime the baby was fussy, Wy was whisked from my arms by one of Michael's parents, who scowled at my inexperience. I didn't think that I had a right to speak up for myself, because I had zero experience as a wife or mother. I also had no husband there to stand up for me. Michael couldn't tolerate being around his neurotic parents for more than a few days. I soon understood why. I realized the reason he went to military school was to get away from them. They made today's worst "helicopter" parents look like amateurs.

Of course, this was not an ideal beginning to a marriage or motherhood, but I was scared to death and unprepared for both and I had nowhere else to go and no money of my own. Later, I saw the Ciminellas as a source of support for both my daughters over the years of their childhoods and young adulthood, and they all had a mutual adoration for one another.

*   *   *

In 1964, at age eighteen, I felt doomed, except for my bond with my newborn daughter. It became the only real relationship in my life. Over time it has remained a partnership that has been the most challenging one of my life and has also brought me the most joy, especially when Wy and I are in sync with each other onstage. It has always given me a feeling of being the most alive. Wynonna and I are like moths, dancing around each other's bright flames. As a singing duo there is always the energy and beauty of the mother-daughter spark between us; yet as individuals, the flammability of our raw emotions can burn. During our final tour together, in 2011, we each came home with singed and damaged wings. The enmeshment we had on the Encore tour became far too intense.

Wy and I had both agreed to allow the new Oprah Winfrey network, OWN, to film a "behind-the-scenes" reality show about the tour. We were honored to be a part of the network's inaugural season on cable. I had never watched this kind of reality show before, where the cameras are with the subject from morning until late night. I truly had no idea what we were signing up to do. The way the OWN producers pitched it to us made it seem like a perfectly reasonable and even fun, by golly, idea. It soon became an overwhelming invasion, with every flicker of emotion followed and encouraged on camera, with the producers asking leading questions meant to get a passionate, uncensored response.

We were taken to places that were certain to bring up unpredictable and raw reactions, emotionally charged locations, such as the Los Angeles house where I had lived in hand-to-mouth poverty, trying to raise Wynonna and Ashley, two very feisty daughters. This was the only place I could afford following my divorce from Michael, who provided no financial support over the years, except for a single check for one hundred dollars.

Wy's memories and perceptions of her time as a child in Los Angeles that she described for the OWN show were difficult and painful for her to express, but feeling very sensitive, I perceived them as accusatory and full of blame. I was going through my own extremely painful emotions, which I was trying to keep internalized, being suddenly taken back to yet another place in my personal history that held long-suppressed trauma of gigantic proportions for me.

All of my memories from those early Los Angeles years in the 1970s were of a breathless struggle to keep us afloat. But that is something a child can't comprehend and I didn't want my daughters to feel the insecurity or grasp the severity of our plight. Wherever we had to drive to in my old beat-up green Impala, I would tell my girls stories or we would sing songs together. I wanted them to know joy, and it was a good distraction from my own mounting worries. Since I had no medical insurance, my greatest fear was that one of us would get sick.

I would pick out all of our clothing at the United Way thrift store and then fold Wy and Ashley's clothes up in a shopping bag, as if they were brand-new. Many meals were bologna, crackers, and canned corn. I told myself it was a balanced meal: meat, vegetable, and a grain.

By the time Wynonna was nineteen, she was beginning to earn a good income from RCA, our recording label, so it was a challenge for her to relate to the desperation of being a single mom and not knowing if you would be living on the street the next month because you fell behind in paying rent. During that week of shooting the OWN show in Los Angeles, I felt exposed and defensive about my necessary past choices and survival methods as a young single mother, even though I had done the best I could.

By our last date of the tour, and once the reality show was wrapped up, Wynonna and I were both emotionally and physically exhausted. We had so many unresolved issues of resentment, anger, and lack of boundaries.

About a week after the finale of the tour, we met with our long-time family therapist, Ted Klontz, at my farm, hoping to resolve any leftover hurt or anger. We both wanted the tour to end on a high note.

Our session was not harmonious. When we tried to discuss anything, even minor problems, the anger flared and became frightening. It was obvious we were living in very different realities. Ted, who has referred to us as "two alpha females in one family," advised us both that when we are so frustrated and emotionally defensive that we might say something we will regret, we should immediately declare "I'm flooded," which means "stop." No explanation required.

It was obvious that we were both drowning. I shut down and so did Wy. After fourteen months of being together daily on the Encore tour, we seemed to be headed for some time apart. I don't think either of us knew how much time.

The day we finished the Encore tour, Larry and I flew home together. In the airport, I took pictures with fans and hugged strangers. I laughed and chatted and told jokes to the airline staff and the flight attendants. It's what I love doing. However, as soon as I sat down on the plane, I felt like my last ounce of energy had been spent. I was taken aback to feel pent-up tears stinging my eyes and spilling out. I wanted to curl against Larry's shoulder and sob, but it wasn't the place. I dabbed at the corners of my eyes with a tissue and then leaned back and pretended to be sleeping. Images flew through my mind of our final bows and the happy faces of the audience looking up at us with warmth and affection. They may have been capturing the moment for their memory books, but so was I. It was the end of an era, an era that I had moved heaven and earth to create.

In the car from the airport, I peered up at the thick layer of clouds hovering over the countryside. It was late October and the air held a damp chilliness that I knew might last until April. A feeling of heavy dread wrapped around me, no matter how hard I tried to shrug it off. I reminded myself that I was physically tired from our nonstop schedule. I was jet-lagged from changing time zones every two days for weeks on end. I thought I was probably going to experience the post-tour blues. I've had the blues before, because I always miss the fans and their joy. I didn't yet suspect that this time was different and that within a week I would wish that I only had the blues.

When I opened the door to my home, I flipped on the light in the hallway. The house was so quiet and seemed so empty. Larry took the dogs and walked to the barn to check on the horses. I could hear the kitchen clock ticking steadily. I had never noticed it in the past. I stood, motionless, listening to the sound of emptiness. At first the clock sounded like a persistent tapping, like someone or something wanting to come in. Then it prodded me like unrelenting questions, demanding my attention, questions that I wanted to ignore, but couldn't. The questions gained entry into my mind and then drilled down to my heart. They terrified me.

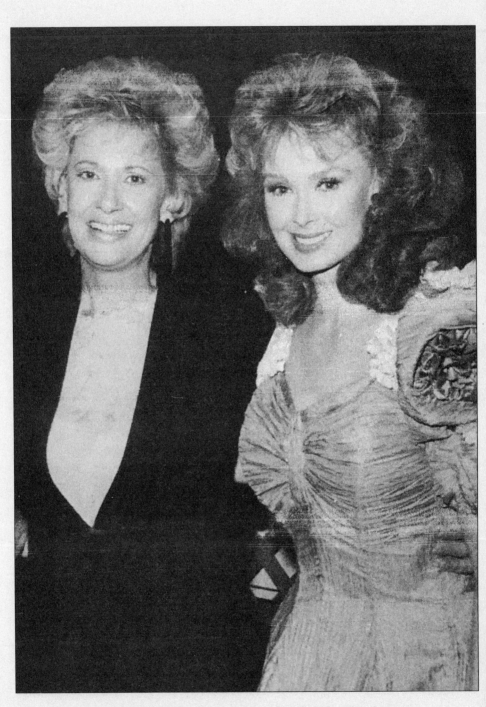

Tammy Wynette became my best friend. She also suffered from deep depression.

Chapter 3

Who Turned Off the Spotlight?

What will be next for you, Naomi? The question I asked myself devastated me. One pesky question followed another. What will you do with yourself tomorrow? What will your days hold next month? What about the rest of your life? Is your time of striving for a career goal completely over? As a harmony singer, becoming a solo act isn't what I want to pursue.

The era of performing before thousands of people has come to a close. There are no more tours set up for the future. There will be no more music publishers knocking on your door for the next song you've written, no fabulous gowns to design, no awards shows to attend, no spotlight shining on the complete joy you feel while onstage. Even your offstage life will never be the same. Your daughters are adults with careers of their own. They don't need you. The grandchildren have grown up and have lives of their own. They don't need you. Your husband is still traveling with his vocal group and is often away. You are on your own now. What in the world are you going to do? Do you have anything to do tomorrow? I tried to shake the questions from my head. I tried to laugh them off as a mock restaurant hostess: "Ms. Judd, pity party of one. Please follow me to your table by the door of doom."

What should have been a welcome home celebration from a successful tour in 2011 felt more like a slow forced march into a bleak future. I was becoming afraid it was the beginning of a descent into darkness I had heard about from other troubled souls who had shared their plight with me.

I had friends who had spoken of being shocked and overwhelmed by similar feelings, women who had dedicated their lives to raising children who were now grown and had moved away. I've known career women who had been laid off or forced to retire before they were ready, or who had husbands whose companies had downsized rapidly. Friends and fans had often told me stories of feeling happy-go-lucky one week and completely unsure and even devastated the next. A friend of mine who works in my town told me that she watched her husband get up every morning and head out the door for his job, as usual. One afternoon, he was spotted alone, reading on a park bench when he should have been at work. This forced him to confess that he had been fired weeks before and was too humiliated to tell his family.

"When you put a lifetime of effort into a career or avocation, what do you do when that focus is gone?" fans and friends would ask me. I could see the fear and uncertainty in their eyes. I listened with sympathy, but I couldn't empathize. I always had the next goal ready to go. The phone continued to ring with more opportunities, so I never slowed down.

I have talked to many women who lost their husbands through death, divorce, or betrayal and were feeling abandoned and alone after giving their best years to a relationship that was now gone. They would tell me that they had fallen into a depression or suffered bouts of anxiety about their futures, confiding that they had no idea who they were now, since they had identified themselves for so many years as a wife, mother, or employee. I'd never seen that as possible in my own future, even though I witnessed as it happened to Mother when Daddy left us.

When my tour bus arrived two days later, wending its way onto our property and to my front door, my only wish was to get on it and be driven away, back to the life I loved and away from the gathering clouds of my darkening mood. Even though the tour had been filled with challenges, every day brought a new city, a different crowd, maybe some unpredictable dilemma or a delightful surprise or two. As long as it was interesting, I felt fully alive and engaged. After all, as a former ICU nurse and with all I've been through, I'm at my best in emergencies.

I couldn't re-create these vibrant feelings anymore since returning home. I tried to take a "back to nature" walk in the valley, something that always refreshed my outlook on life in the past. However, this time the trees seemed looming and threatening.

I attempted to cook a big family meal, which has always brought me pleasure, a connection to my family, evoking a feeling of warmth in the past. This time, though, I had no desire for food. Nothing appealed to me and I began to lose weight. I felt drained of all desires to do anything at all. My mind was repeatedly nudging me, taunting me like a bully: "What's the point, Naomi? Is the rest of your life going to be another walk in the woods, another homemade meal that is eaten and forgotten in twenty minutes? Is that all your future will be?"

The bus driver took my hand to help me climb the steps into the coach. I gave him a hug and smiled, resisting my impulse to say, "Start the engine. We're out of here. I'm not ready to stop. I don't want to be alone with my thoughts." However, "my" bus hadn't arrived to take me somewhere new; it was there to leave me behind. It was time for me to clean out my personal belongings. There would be another touring country singer who would soon be leasing this bus and crisscrossing the country. It was no longer my traveling home.

I made my way to the back of the bus, to my cozy bedroom where I had slept soundly for eleven months. The hum of the massive tires on the highway beneath me and the soft pull of forward motion would lull me to sleep quickly. If I didn't feel especially tired following a concert and a meet-and-greet, after the OWN camera people had called it quits for the day I would make a bag of microwave popcorn and sit in the big captain's chair next to the bus driver and we'd talk and look out at the starry night, like pilgrims on a journey into uncharted territory. There is something so simply relaxing about knowing that your only goal for the next ten or twelve hours is to let the driver take you to the next city on the tour.

Since the mid-1980s, when Wynonna and I went on our first national tour, I have always been most "at home" on a tour bus. I'm happy having a zip code–free life. We would arrive in a city, park in back of the venue near the stage door, do a sound check, have dinner with the crew, do a two-hour show, meet with our fans for hours after the performance, then get on our bus and watch a movie, tell funny stories, share a homemade cake or treats from a fan, and eat bag after bag of microwave popcorn.

When we first started out, it was a more intimate setting, with the band in bunks near the front of the bus and Wynonna and me with small bedrooms in the back. It was like having a close-knit family without the complications of actually being family. We would go to bed at two in the morning in the Black Hills of South Dakota and wake up nine hours later at the Red Rocks amphitheater in Colorado.

After so many years of struggling along as a single mother, trying to piece together a way to support my children while living in a series of dilapidated apartment buildings, broken-down cabins, roach-infested hotel rooms, and drafty rented houses, I welcomed the chance to live in our clean, comfortable little house on wheels. Even though I now own a lovely home, the tour bus life still holds its charm.

For the Encore tour, Wy and I each had our own bus, and the band had a bus, too, which seemed like quite a luxury compared to our past. We would travel caravan-style, along with six more buses carrying the crew, band, instruments, and stage set, winding our way across the United States. I was completely content, and proud of our visible success.

There are certain items I take with me on every road trip or tour to make myself feel at home. I always look forward to arranging them around me in any new situation. Now it was time to pack them up.

I tugged my favorite quilt from the top of the bed, folding it into a box along with my most comfortable flannel pj's with the monkey faces design that Wynonna had given me. On my bedside stand were the framed photos I always keep nearby, both of family. Next to that was my little box with my trusty earplugs and eyedrops, alongside a bottle of eucalyptus oil that I always keep nearby for aromatherapy. I had left some of my favorite books on the bus, a few of the gifts the fans had given me, and my cosmetics bag, all of which I put in the box. On the shelf near the door was where I had placed a beautiful natural violet and blue crystal geode stone, about the size of a grapefruit, an amethyst, given to me by a Native American friend, who always regales me with fascinating stories of natural healings.

Amethyst stones have been treasured for centuries and are believed to have a calming and positive effect. I use it as a meditative stone for emotional balance and peaceful thoughts. I told him that I would take it on the tour as my "altar." Whenever I needed to "alter" my frame of mind to be more positive, I would gaze at that geode.

I opened the closet door to my gorgeous stage costumes. A reporter once asked me why I didn't dress more casual country and wear jeans and cowgirl boots for the shows. I gave her a double answer. First, I've never owned cowgirl boots or a pair of blue jeans; they're not my style. Second, I've always wanted the audience to have a "wow" experience both musically and visually. I knew that it was expensive for many of them to buy tickets, pay for babysitters, drive into the city, and park, all to see our show. I knew that our concert was a two-hour vacation they could take away from their own worries and troubles. If I could fit more sparkle and bling, another rhinestone or dyed feather on my gowns, it would certainly be there. It made me feel glamorous and I passed that good feeling of self-confidence on to the audience.

As I took the dresses off the hangers, I wondered if I should just put them in a bag and give them to someone who could use them. Or, perhaps the fans would like to have them. After all, I would never have the opportunity to wear them again. The concerts were behind me now. Still, it seemed inconceivable that I would never tour by bus again. The magical journey had ended. Someone had turned the spotlight out.

Now, as the empty tour bus turned to lumber back down our long driveway toward the main road, I stood alone, watching it go, as the bitterly cold wind lashed my hair across my face and rattled the cardboard box in my arms. I couldn't even try to hold back the tears. I wasn't sure I could make it back into the house. I felt as though the joy that the world had given me so much of through performing for the past year had evaporated before my eyes, leaving me a deflated woman without any sense of purpose. It's said that when you leave Shangri-la, you turn old and gray. I had lost my identity.

When I finally made my way back inside, I crumbled onto the kitchen couch in the same way marathon runners sometimes collapse after the finish line. I was emotionally exhausted. I don't know how long I sat there, except I remember it going from daylight outside to a pitch-black, moonless night. I didn't turn on a light, but I did turn on the TV. I found an old episode of *Law & Order.* I scrolled through the cable guide and saw there was a nonstop string of *Law & Order* reruns all evening. Without even getting up for a drink of water, I put my feet up on the box I had packed on the bus and watched one episode after another until Larry got home from his rehearsal. He wanted to know why I was sitting in complete darkness. I would have answered him, but I had no explanation. So I muttered, "Shhh. Chief Dodd is telling Benson to expect changes. It doesn't look good."

Larry put on the kitchen lights so he could see my face. He looked at me in silence for a minute. It seemed as if the plot I had described might be playing out in my real life. Expect changes, Naomi Judd. And it doesn't look good.

A few days later, I still didn't have the energy or ambition to unpack. My costumes lay bunched up across the upstairs railing, my stage shoes were scattered on the floor, and I had kicked the cardboard box to the side of the kitchen couch. This was not like me at all. Larry called our longtime friend and part-time house manager, Angie, to come over and help to straighten up our disorganized home. She is a true southern gal. I could see the shock on her face when she saw me again. Angie took one look at me and proclaimed,

"You are in a bad way, girlfriend." I supervised what needed to happen from the couch, apologizing between my tears that I couldn't help her. Angie gently hugged me and set a box of tissues nearby.

Larry encouraged me to have some social interaction, to meet up with a friend or two in our village at a café, hoping I would abandon my protective nest on the couch, but I had no interest in doing anything. I didn't have enough energy to be out in public and I certainly didn't want anyone to know I was sinking deeper day by day into despair.

From spending years on the road, the women I considered my friends were my fellow performers. I felt very fortunate to have been on the country music scene with a generation of women artists who were kind, funny, and generous enough to extend a hand of friendship to newcomers. The one-of-a-kind Dolly Parton became my friend. I share a bond with Reba McIntyre, and we have spent time at each other's homes. Martina McBride and I developed a friendship and she also has visited me. In turn, I was thrilled to see the quality of upcoming talent like Carrie Underwood, who fell in love with the property where I live in Tennessee. I sold a few of my acres to her so she could build her own family home and become my neighbor.

Undoubtedly, my best friend in the country music world was Tammy Wynette. She and I shared a common small-town history: divorce, moving to Nashville with children in tow and not a penny to our names, having a golden opportunity to audition for a record producer in person, and then having preposterous dreams become a fabulous reality. We recognized our bond the day we met. After that, we would talk a few times a week on the phone at night, before she would go to bed at nine thirty. She had chronic pain from many health issues and more than twenty-six different surgeries and was addicted to strong painkillers, even though she had bravely sought treatment for the addiction at the Betty Ford Center.

I believe Tammy was a victim of the trust she placed in her last husband, George Richey, to take care of her and make sure her medications and dosages were correct. It seems her faith in her twenty-year marriage was misplaced and it cost Tammy her life.

On a chilly spring night, Richey called our house at 1 a.m. He told me that Tammy was in the ICU at Baptist Hospital in Nashville and was "really bad off." She was asking to see me. Still in my pj's, I broke the speed limit getting to the hospital that night. She could barely speak, but I lowered the bed rail and crawled in to lie beside her and hold her hand. Some days later, after returning home, she died on her own couch from an overdose of painkillers.

You can read for yourselves the public opinions of Tammy's children and their suspicions about George Richey's role in their mother's death. Even though the lawsuit against him was eventually dropped, I stand by Tammy's three girls. They knew their mother was in trouble but felt helpless because she was vulnerable to the will of her husband, who was infatuated with and then married Tammy's "personal secretary," a woman who had tried to befriend Wynonna and me, appearing by our tour bus after shows. I never liked her and always felt a deep suspicion about her motives.

Legendary Tammy Wynette left us at age fifty-five, but I feel, in my heart, she would be here still if she had been under someone else's care. I often think of Tammy and wonder, if she had had more close friends watching out for her, whether her story would have ended so tragically. One of the most prophetic things Tammy said about her own life's tribulations was "The sad part about happy endings is there's nothing to write about."

I still longed for my own happy ending. I saw the wisdom in Larry's suggestion about social interaction. I agreed it would boost my chances to return to a happier life if I established a circle of women friends. My village is full of interesting and lively women and I decided it was time to make an effort to form friendships with some of them. I invited a number of likable women I had met in recent years to come over for an evening get-together. Two women are accomplished oil painters who sell very well; another runs the village newspaper. I invited a professional photographer and a backup singer, along with an interior decorator and a store owner. The small group also included women who owned a yoga studio and a landscaping business, and two wise women who have mastered life's vicissitudes. I didn't explain much about the gathering in the invitation, except I that I hoped to establish a group bond, like the one in the movie *The Divine Secrets of the Ya-Ya Sisterhood*. I asked all of them to wear clothing that flowed and I dressed up in a Mother Nature costume with flowers and small branches and leaves in my hair.

We gathered in the "great room" of my house, where I had a roaring fire in the massive stone fireplace and finger food snacks. Besides asking them to dress a certain way, the only other thing I requested was for each woman to bring a picture of herself at age ten. We sat in a circle and I asked each of them to share with the rest of the group what their hopes and dreams were at age ten and what they felt about those dreams today. There were quite a few laughs and even some tears as the women recalled their ambitions and their disappointments.

I studied the picture of myself at age ten. I was a child who was very likely to strike a pose, hands on hips, with a movie star tilt to my head. I dreamed of a colorful and expressive lifestyle, much different from the one in which I was being raised. I didn't know how

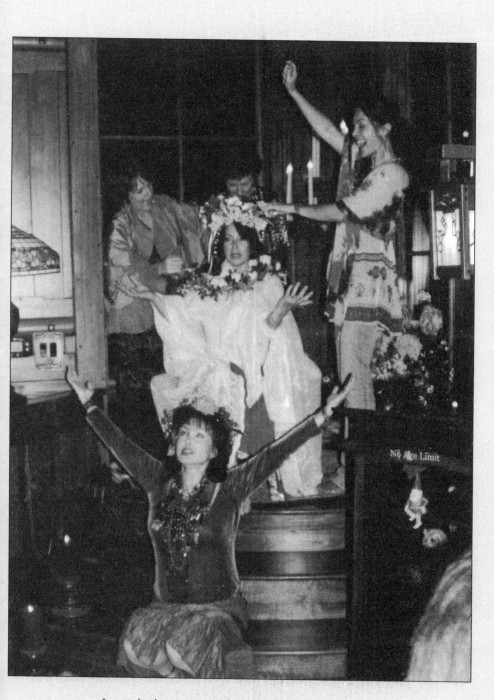

I wanted to have a group of close girlfriends so this was our first
Divine Secrets of the Ya-Ya Sisterhood–*type ceremony.*

I would achieve my dreams at the time. I only knew I had to, somehow, survive. The other women commented on my determination and courage in achieving all I had. I tried to joke by saying that "we all have days when the toilet backs up, and I discovered, years ago, you have to have a plunger and learn how to turn off the water."

Even if I appeared successful to my new friends, I could no longer feel the pride I once had in my accomplishments. The little girl in the photo was still in me, but her hands-on-hips defiance wasn't going to work in dealing with the emotional pain I was experiencing.

After hearing my story, the women declared that my new spiritual sisterhood name would be "Wisdom Seeker." Each of the other women was given a new sisterhood name such as "High Priestess" and "Grand Poo-bah" as they ceremoniously rode the elevator down from my second floor and made an entrance into the great room. I passed out oversized colorful scarves that we ceremoniously wrapped around our shoulders. I had everyone jump to her feet as I thumped out a rhythm on a set of Native American drums Larry keeps in his recording studio. We danced with great abandon, like happy kids, holding our scarves over our heads.

It was the best I had felt since returning home from the tour. I was surprised and touched at how willing these women were to play along. Our inner child had definitely come out to play. At the end of the night, we hugged and pledged our sisterhood to each other in good times and in bad. We shared our phone numbers and set up a chain reaction phone grid for whoever needed help. One sister would phone the next and down the line to arrange a time and place to meet for the sister who was in need. We all agreed on the significance of having a female support system.

Larry seemed enormously relieved by my contented mood when we went to bed that night and was hoping that my blues had waned. I was feeling pleased that my sisterhood idea had worked out so beautifully. As I dozed off I was planning a second get-together in my head. Four hours later, I was jolted awake, feeling as if someone had dumped stinging wasps all over my arms, face, and neck. I couldn't breathe in deeply. My heart was racing with adrenaline. I shook Larry's shoulder and told him that something was really wrong. He checked my face and arms and said they looked fine. He tried to help me to calm my breathing by having me inhale more slowly. I burst into anxious tears, feeling I was about to die. Larry put his arm around me, but I couldn't stay still. I had to get up and pace. After three or four hours of walking the floors, I could finally sit down once I saw that dawn was breaking over the horse pasture.

Later that morning, one of the women called me to say what a great time she had. She was so happy to have this new group of friends. I tried to respond with enthusiasm, but it had drained away after the hours of anxiety. It was now apparent to me that no amount of playacting or sorority atmosphere was going to ward off my painful memories or the persisting anxiety. No dancing with abandon to a drumbeat could control my pounding heart during a panic attack.

I began sinking deeper and deeper into despair over the following days. The only thing that felt almost as bad as the depression was the tremendous shame about it. After all, I was living the life many people dream of having: international fame, a great marriage, wonderful friends, and a gorgeous farm with acres of property. I had authored bestselling books and shared my ideas on how to live a happy and optimistic life. I was especially convincing on how a woman can feel great as she ages.

I felt like a fraud. I had now gone for more than three weeks without putting on makeup and barely brushing my hair. I would change out of one pair of pajamas and into another, never putting on regular clothes. I rambled through the days in exhaustion from countless sleepless nights and tear-filled hours of emotional and physical pain. In the morning, I might manage to make it downstairs for a cup of coffee. That alone would make me feel exhausted, so I would lie down on the couch and stay there for hours. Larry started to bring in carryout food, since I wasn't looking in the refrigerator. I couldn't even seem to find the initiative to make toast in the morning. I would leave the carryout food untouched and surf the TV channels, hoping to find yet another episode of *Law & Order.* There was something in the dramatic events of that show that took me away from the prison of my own thoughts.

Every evening, as I was brushing my teeth before bed, I would feel the anticipation of another nightmarish panic attack happening again after just a few hours of sleep. Though I tried to ignore it, the fear would seep into my thoughts.

Larry and I would try to watch a fun late-night show together from our bed. He would hold my hand tightly, but eventually he would doze off and I would feel his hand go limp in mine. Then my trepidations would kick up to high intensity. Would it happen again? The fear of the panic attack became a self-fulfilling prophecy. The more distress I felt at the possibility of panic, the more it completely consumed me. I believed I was the only person on earth who had ever had panic attacks this bad for so many days.

Chapter 4
Potato Salad on the Hood of the Car

After one long night of walking the floors with my heart racing and gasping for a full breath, I huddled on the kitchen couch in the dark, where Larry found me. He sat down next to me and told me he had something on his mind, something that had been building up for a while. I looked into his eyes, which seemed full of defeat. This is it, I thought. My misery is driving him away for good. Is he leaving me?

"I don't recognize you anymore," Larry confessed. "I don't know how to help you." He held my hands in his and made me look him in the eye. I didn't want to hear what he would say next. I held my breath as the worst-case scenario raced through my head. If he tells me he's leaving, then what? I'll be alone. I've always been terrified of being alone. It's my greatest fear.

Larry's voice stayed firm and calm, "You've had a complete personality change. You've got to get serious professional help."

I wasn't sure whether to feel relief or anger. There was comfort in knowing that he would stay with me. And then I felt a deep concern that my own husband was telling me that I was losing my mind. Was he right? We trust each other implicitly. Was this how it would

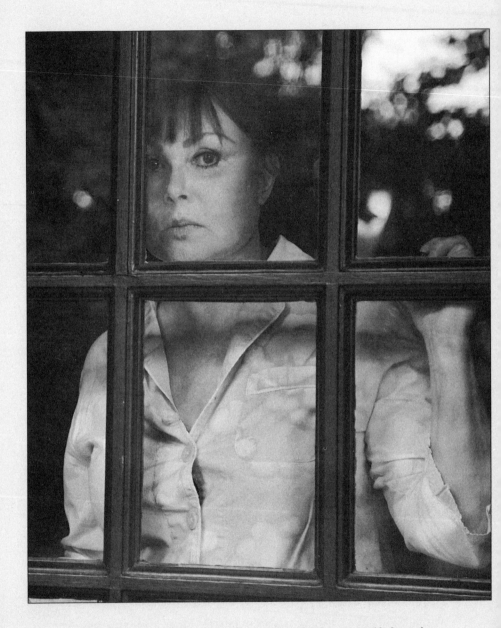

My beautiful farm became my prison. Sometimes I didn't step outside for weeks.

be now? Was this depression driving me crazy? I wasn't ready to admit defeat, even though I could no longer recognize myself, either.

I tried to convince Larry that it was a passing phase, caused by the trauma of losing my career, and I would soon be myself again. I reminded him that I had trained and worked for years as a nurse and I would certainly know if I needed professional help. I had been around many patients who suffered from all types of maladies. I could tell Larry had serious doubts, and I was trying my best to pull off some good acting, since my own doubts were at least twice as strong as his.

I was known for surviving the death sentence decreed upon me by specialists in hepatitis C treatment. My attitude was, "Oh yeah? I'll show you." I determined that I would find the answer to my predicament, and find it naturally, mind over matter.

Now it seemed my mind had taken over the matter in my brain in ways that were becoming uncontrollable. But I wasn't ready to wave the white flag. I was still convinced that I could fight depression on my own and had no idea that struggling with this serious illness without medication and other help would lead to what is known as "panic disorder."

The holidays were approaching, but my usual festive spirit was nowhere to be seen. My daughter Ashley was completely devoted to her ongoing worldwide humanitarian work and she was often traveling out of the country. When she called from foreign countries, I would control my voice to sound as normal as possible. I was glad she couldn't see my face. Wynonna seemed to be 100 percent wrapped up in her exciting dating life with her new boyfriend Cactus and blending the lives of their teenagers. I knew she was booking concert dates for 2012, and was busy resuming her solo career on the road and in the studio. I had not heard her beautiful voice in what seemed like a terribly long time. My days seemed to grow longer. I anticipated that I would soon be myself once again, yet, in truth, I felt like I was falling into a dark, endless abyss, alone. I didn't attempt to connect with Wynonna, because I had no words for what was happening to me or why. How could I explain it when I was becoming a stranger to myself? In my vulnerability, I wanted her to reach out to me first, but I also wanted to give her the space to process for herself. My emotions were multilayered and complicated. As Wynonna clearly stated in her January 2015 televised interview with Dan Rather, who asked her about her family relationships, she was tired of being "reactive instead of proactive." In retrospect, it appears that "proactive" in Wy's definition meant that she couldn't be around those she felt "reactive" to, which would be me.

One chilly December afternoon, my well-meaning group of sisterhood girlfriends convinced me to go antiquing with them. I could barely generate a single ounce of enthusiasm about the excursion. I was as uptight as a banjo string. Still, I had the thought that it would help to foster Larry's hope that I would soon be back to acting like my ol' self again. I could see an increasing shadow of worry on his face.

He has told me many times that one of the reasons he fell in love with me more than thirty-seven years ago was that I always knew what I wanted to do and how to get it done. That seemed to be one of my character traits that resonated with almost every person in my life. When Wynonna and I toured almost continuously between 1984 and 1991, I was the decision maker. I would almost look forward to the next challenge. Everyone from the bus driver to the backstage crew would turn to me to solve problems, from what to do for an earache to how to handle a technical emergency like the sound board blowing up.

A sliver of raw garlic clove wrapped in tissue would solve the earache and a call to the musicians' union, which answers 24/7, would give us access to someone who could replace the sound board within an hour or two. I took every complication in stride. My coworkers and family have always been more than willing to let me take charge. They nicknamed me "the Queen of Serene." But now I could not figure out how to fix my deepening depression and panic attacks and it was really starting to scare me.

I stood for fifteen minutes before my open closet door, paralyzed. I was unable to choose what to wear for an afternoon of shopping with the girls. I finally found a pair of black stretch pants and a jacket that I could zip up over a T-shirt, an outfit that I would normally never wear for an afternoon outing in town, but it was the best decision I could manage. I pulled my hair back into a rough twist and pushed it under a newsboy wool cap. I applied a heavy layer of cover stick makeup over the dark circles under my eyes.

At the first antique store, I wandered around, listening to the other women laugh and talk. I turned the corner, around a tall white armoire, and looked directly into an antique mirror in a gilded frame. The frame was ornate, but the mirror had about a dozen cracks running through it in jagged lines. The reflection of my face in the mirror, divided and distorted into broken pieces, stopped me cold. My image resembled exactly how I felt inside, jagged pieces, barely held together. I had a sinking feeling that this crazed reflection was symbolic not only of my present, but of my future.

*   *   *

The holidays came and went in a blur. I ventured out to buy a few gifts for the family and it took every bit of energy I could muster.

Every year, Larry and I throw a huge Christmas party at our house, a holiday gala that takes weeks of preparation. Our friends and family look forward to this gathering. I usually start talking about it in early October. Some of our friends even count this warm and intimate evening as their Christmas. One couple, Gary and Alex, retail gift shop owners, don't put up a single decoration in their own home, because they get such a large dose of Christmas at my house. Every banister, door frame, nook, and corner in my house is decorated, even to the point of poinsettia plants and candles in the bathroom!

We invite about ninety people and have a catered buffet, an open bar with a bartender, and tables and chairs set up strategically throughout the entire downstairs where people can gather, eat, and chat. In our great room we arrange a stage area for live entertainment near the massive stone fireplace. There is always a keyboard player, drums, and guitars. Before the evening ends, we all gather around the piano to sing Christmas carols from old-fashioned songbooks.

As a child, I always dreamed of cozy, warm family gatherings like the ones portrayed on the covers of Christmas catalogs. I would picture scenes of pine boughs strung across our fireplace mantel with lit candles and angel figurines nestled in between. In my fantasies, there was a beautiful holy manger scene on a red and green table runner, candy canes and a plate of frosted cookies for Santa, and a stack of Christmas records playing continuously on our hi-fi. That's not how it was, in the least. It was only near the front window of the living room that it looked like Christmas at all at our house. We would have a tree with sparse ornaments set up there, some handmade from our Sunday school classes.

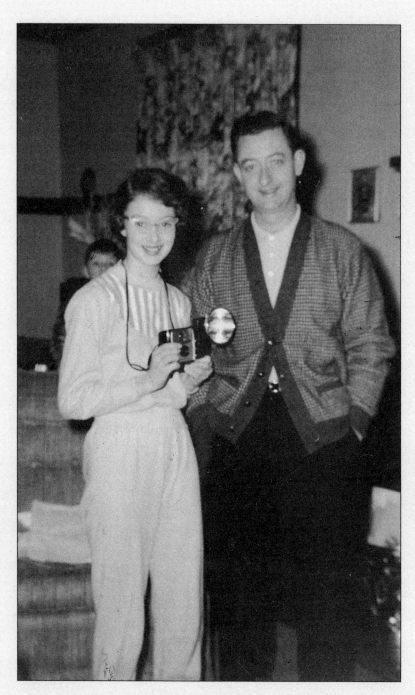

I loved my daddy. This Christmas when I was fifteen,
I got a camera and he got a sweater.

We had no Christmas music, only one Tennessee Ernie Ford album of church hymns. I longed to have Daddy read "'Twas the Night Before Christmas" or sing "Jingle Bells" with us. I wanted my grandparents and aunts to ask me what I wanted for Christmas, but no one ever did. And no gifts were ever given. Santa usually brought a few gifts for my siblings and me.

When I was ten, my Santa wish list was the boldest one yet. I wanted a bicycle. The other girls at my elementary school had all been given brand-new bikes for their seventh or eighth birthdays, but my ninth and then tenth birthday came and went with no bike to ride. So eleven months later I wrote it down as my only gift request from Santa.

On Christmas morning, I was beyond excited. I rushed down the stairs and Daddy pointed to the front door. There was a blue Schwinn bike on the front porch. Santa had paid attention to me! I sprinted toward the shiny handlebars. But they weren't as shiny up close and the handgrips were stained and cracked. The white rims of the tires were more of a dingy gray and there was a long scratch right in the middle of the frame near the pedals. This couldn't be from Santa. He would never bring a used bike, especially to a little girl who tried so hard to be good and made certain she had a perfect report card. I looked over at Daddy's face but he lit one of his unfiltered Camel cigarettes and turned away. My siblings were unwrapping their presents and Mother had gone to the kitchen to make coffee.

Three of my childhood beliefs were destroyed in that one moment. Any lingering belief in a Santa Claus was gone. My dream of a perfect family Christmas was smashed. And, most damaging for me, my feeling of basic security was jeopardized. My ten-year-old mind scrambled to understand what this battered old bike represented. We must be poor. Something must have happened and no one is saying anything. What would happen to us? I was terrified.

As extreme as my thought process was that Christmas Day, it was strongly reinforced when neither one of my parents would come outside to teach me to ride the bike. Were they both ashamed of the used bike?

As I struggled to learn to balance and pedal without training wheels, my emotions teetered back and forth from the feelings of betrayal to the reminder of my resolve that I would figure out my own way to take care of myself. That would become the pattern of how my life would progress: free-falling into each new experience with no training wheels to keep me from a painful spill, but always figuring out a way to get wherever I wanted to go.

Once Larry and I moved into our beautiful house on our farm in Tennessee, I knew I could create the kind of merry Christmas I had always wanted. I made sure that my friends were able to have that magical holiday, too. This year, though, for the first time, I had a nervous apprehension about hosting the party. Would they notice that I was not myself? Would they wonder what was happening to me? I felt as if I were watching the festivities from a distance and not really there. I fought back tears. People would hug me and try to talk to me and I did my best to respond, but I couldn't even keep up a cheerful conversation. I was the Ghost of Christmas Past, dragging heavy chains of unresolved PTSD. Even to "sleep in heavenly peace" had become an impossibility.

Ashley was back in town for Christmas week, after a long humanitarian trip to work with children in Africa, and came over in a jovial holiday mood. She wondered why I wasn't cooking as

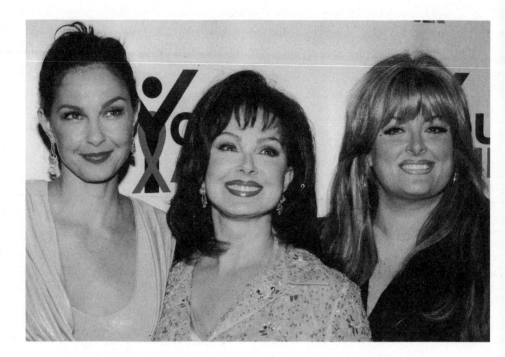

much as I usually did, but I shrugged it off by saying I was still tired from the tour. Wynonna came over later on Christmas Day, after celebrating with Cactus and the kids in the morning, and we exchanged our gifts. But we didn't have a chance to exchange much in the way of words as the house filled with family and the meal was being prepared.

Because we spent so much time together on the road over the years, I know Wy's taste in clothes and accessories and she, in turn, knows mine. The gift I bought her made her smile and that made me feel good, but she left the beautiful long coat at my house, not taking it with her, as if to say she didn't want "things," she wanted understanding. Even though it wasn't the right time to talk, seeing her face I remembered that we are still bonded for life, no matter what.

On New Year's Eve, I was in bed at 8 p.m. I halfheartedly prayed that I would have a new start with the New Year, while not really caring if I woke up to see even one day of 2012.

Every January 1, I start a brand-new Day-Timer planner. I have always chronicled my life, day by day, making notes of how I felt and interactions with new people I met. My journal for 2011 has a full list of experiences on almost every date before November, when I had returned from the tour. In 2012, my first three months show that I spent almost every single day on the couch in my kitchen. I attended very few functions or social events and then only made a brief appearance and came up with an excuse to leave after a few minutes. Larry no longer believed my story that this was "just a phase." Neither did I.

The mornings were quickly becoming as unbearable as the nighttime. I was to find out later that depression tends to be worse in the mornings. Even if I had been able to fall asleep the night before, I would wake up with a jolt at 3 a.m. My nighttime panic attacks were so frequent now that I would do my best to not wake Larry up anymore. He was becoming exhausted from his own interrupted sleep. Once the panic subsided, the depression would wrap me in a heavy cloak of despair. It seemed that the panic disorder and lasting depression were trying to bury me alive. Worse still was that I was beginning not to care if my life ended. The only thing I cared about was disappointing my family, who always looked to me to be the steadfast matriarch.

Larry and I have a small group of close friends, three other couples, of more than twenty years called "the Unusual Suspects." We try to gather for a potluck dinner at one of our houses at least once a month, and then watch movies or play games, like charades. These are fun-loving, intelligent, caring, good-hearted people. We all know each other and our families so well. I looked forward to our get-togethers and my friends referred to me as "the life of the party." I certainly didn't fit that description anymore. I rarely smiled for days on end. I moved slowly and my sense of balance was off.

As 2012 progressed, I could tell that I was devolving, day by day, and hour by hour, into a stumbling zombie. My usually perky personality seemed to be circling the drain. I would tell the other "Suspects" that I would attend the upcoming potluck dinner, but then I would feel a burdensome dread descend on me. I couldn't bear to face anyone anymore, including my best friends. I started backing out of all of our social engagements. I would still make the food that I had promised to bring, but I would leave it on top of my car in the driveway for one of the "Suspects" to pick up.

Even if they knocked on the door to check on me, I wouldn't answer it. I'd hide behind the curtain. It didn't take my friends long to understand that if the big yellow bowl of my famous potato salad was waiting for them to pick up on top of my car, then I was truly not well. I would, again, retreat to the security of the kitchen couch and stare blankly at the cast of strangers who had no expectations of me: the characters on *NCIS* or *Law & Order* reruns.

I had begged Larry not to tell our friends about what was going on with me. I especially made him promise to not talk about my depression or anxiety with Ashley or Wynonna. As a result, my depressed state of mind left me feeling more isolated than I had ever felt in my life.

In the late spring of 2012, Larry once again pulled a chair up to the kitchen couch and sat with his head bowed and his eyes focused on his hands in his lap. There would be no more convincing him that I would bounce back soon. I knew it and Larry knew it. It was time to seek the help of a professional. Truthfully, it was long past time. I had now become a danger to myself.

My thoughts were in such disarray that I couldn't possibly have good judgment in choosing a therapist. But I was determined to keep my depression as my secret, so I didn't ask anyone for recommendations to help me find a highly qualified doctor. I blindly trusted that a run-of-the-mill Nashville psychiatrist I had met at one event in the past year would understand the complexities of the neurochemical brainstorm in my head. He ran me through a number of tests and then told me that he had determined from the results that I had both severe treatment-resistant depression and extreme anxiety.

What I didn't know then is that there are many types of depression, and knowledge about the illness is crucial when it comes to prescribing the right medications. I thought this man with a medical degree in psychiatry would know what he was doing. I didn't expect to be his "trial and error" guinea pig.

He decided to put me on SSRIs (selective serotonin reuptake inhibitors), or what are called antidepressants. Serotonin is the feel-good chemical that our brains should produce naturally. For twenty million Americans, that doesn't happen in the quantity that it should. *Reuptake* is the word that describes the process that is altered by the drug. Instead of the serotonin being absorbed back into the body, the SSRI should cause the serotonin to stay in the brain longer, increasing the feeling of well-being.

Larry and I drove back to the farm with a sense of optimism. Perhaps these prescription drugs I held in my hand would be the simple answer. Could it be that my brain only needed a bit of medicinal support? I was ready to try anything. But, ominously, like a harbinger of the future, when we pulled onto the highway, a bank of dark clouds blew in and a chilling downpour pelted the car all the way home.

After three weeks on Zoloft and Lexapro, I felt like a new person. But not a person anyone would ever want to get to know.

Chapter 5

One Pill Makes You Larger
and One Pill Makes You Small

I was not allowed to slam a door when I was a teenager. I never really thought about doing it, because I knew it would result in punishment once Daddy got home. But now, three weeks into taking an antidepressant, I was so agitated that I found myself slamming doors in my own house, even when I wasn't intending to. The least little thing would infuriate me to the point where I couldn't hide it. If I were home, I'd go upstairs and into the bedroom, where Larry couldn't hear me. I'd let loose with a five-minute string of four-letter words and leave fist dents in every pillow on the bed.

If I went out in the car to run a short errand, I would find myself leaning on the horn and flipping off other drivers who took my parking spot. I got quite a few incredulous stares from other drivers and their passengers. I know they were thinking, Is that Naomi Judd flipping me the bird? They would have been twice as surprised to realize I was carrying a titanium baseball bat and a gun in my car.

I couldn't concentrate or focus my attention for more than a few minutes. I could tell that it was getting harder for even Larry to be around me. My standard answer to his every question was, "Later. I'll deal with it later."

We have done family counseling over the years and have learned good interaction skills, which Larry and I usually applied to any issue. For example, if Larry wanted to talk about the credit card bill, I could have the option of saying, "I'm not in a place to discuss that right now." Through our past therapy, Larry would know to respond: "Okay, I hear you. I accept that. When can we talk about it?" That would allow me the freedom to say something like, "Let's talk in an hour." Larry was trying to continue using this method of communicating, but each time I would reschedule the discussion. Then, when the new time would come, I'd tell him, "I'm not clear-headed. I can't talk to you now."

After three weeks of this, he realized that the chance to talk about anything involving my mental state was not going to happen. My nerves were more on edge than they had been when Wynonna and I performed at Super Bowl halftime for 72,000 people in the Georgia Dome and millions around the world. That was exciting. This was excruciating. My depression grew deeper than it was before I started medication and my anxiety increased with each passing night.

After a month, Larry drove me back to see the Nashville psychiatrist. I don't know why I never questioned that this doctor did zero follow-up or any talk therapy with me after giving me the first prescription. I've had doctors show more concern about how I was doing after something as simple as an eye exam. He never even suggested that I start some talk therapy with someone else; instead, he wrote the third prescription and sent me on my way feeling more confused than comforted.

I explained my worsening condition as best as I could and then the psychiatrist reassured me that even if these current SSRIs weren't helping, there were many others to try. I left with different prescriptions in hand and was told to stop taking the first ones I'd been given and start the new prescriptions as soon as possible. I never questioned his advice. I trusted that this well-dressed professional in his nice office with a wall full of degrees knew what he was doing.

Weeks later I was in a progressively worse state of mind. The third prescription had even less effect in lifting my depression than the first two and had done nothing but increase my anger and feeling of hopelessness. The Nashville psychiatrist called in yet another SSRI prescription, explaining to me that he would, eventually, land on the one that helped.

That night, as I lay in bed, dreading the feeling of anxiety that was percolating under my breastbone, unbidden memories arose of my brother Brian and one of the last few hours I spent with him before he died a slow and terrible death. Brian was in the hospital in Columbus, Ohio, and my parents had agreed to let me go with them to visit him. They had always gone by themselves and had never given me a clue as to what was wrong with him.

We checked in to a dingy, run-down tourist home on the outskirts of Columbus and headed over to the hospital. I didn't want to go back to that awful, moldy room with my parents at the end of the day, so I told them I would sit up in Brian's hospital room overnight. It had been a long time since I had had any time alone with my best childhood buddy.

Brian stayed awake as much as he could to talk with me. I told him stories of everything that was happening in Ashland, which didn't take much time. We talked about our days of playing cowboy and cowgirl, in our little felt hats with the string pulled tight under the chin. We recalled boosting each other up on a wooden soda bottle box to be tall enough to play the pinball machine at Daddy's gas station, and trying to look up high on the shelves where the cartoon-style "girl in a bikini" car air fresheners were stored, out of the sight line of children. We laughed about how risqué that seemed to our young eyes. We talked about TV shows we watched together, never missing a *Twilight Zone* episode.

When Brian started to tire, I helped him adjust his pillows and lowered the hospital bed, so he could lie down. He looked at me for a moment and then asked poignantly, "Am I dying? No one will tell me what's going on."

His question took my breath away. I mumbled, "I don't want you to. So, don't." A flash of a grin moved across his face in the same way it happens on the lips of a sleeping infant. The rest of the night, I sat in my little metal chair with my forehead on the edge of his bedcovers and wept. I couldn't imagine my life without my good-humored, redheaded brother. After spending these precious hours with him, I knew this might be the last time I would ever see him.

In the hallways of the hospital, I could hear other children and teenagers whimpering in pain, or crying out for their parents or a nurse. Some of the nurses who came in during that night to check on my sleeping brother seemed rushed and exhausted, but others were warm and compassionate.

The nurses came to work, every day, in a place where the children were hurting or scared. They had to handle worried family members, look them in the face, and explain both good news and bad news. The nurse is often a buffer between the doctor's diagnosis and how a patient and his family receive the news. If a nurse can't give hope, they can at least give comfort. It was the first time I had seen what a respectable and helpful career nursing could be. Watching these nurses on that sad night made such an impression on me that, years later, I adopted their best characteristics in my own approach to my career as a nurse.

Subsequently, I was appalled by the lack of compassion that came with my own diagnosis of hepatitis C. I'll never forget the distant and impersonal look on the doctor's face when he showed me the results of my liver biopsy. Even though I had already been through nurses' training, had my degree, and had worked for five years as an RN, hepatitis C had not yet been formally defined, so I didn't recognize the symptoms. In 1989, the doctors could only use the term "non-A, non-B," because scientists didn't yet know how to identify this virus.

I was busy taping a Christmas special with Bob Hope when I began to feel extremely exhausted and decided to see the doctor. I expected I would be told I had a resistant bacterial infection that was making me feel like I had the flu every day. Truthfully, though, I had not felt well for three years, and I was pushing out of my mind the fact that as time passed it was getting worse instead of better. I assumed it was the pace of touring and performing live concerts, almost daily press interviews, and TV shows.

When the doctor informed me that I had the hepatitis C virus and that my liver was on the brink of cirrhosis, I thought he must have been reading the wrong chart. Now, twenty-five years later, there has been tremendous treatment progress and a successful oral cure developed that is working for many. But in 1990, my diagnosis was grim, with no hope of a cure. With the same tone of voice as someone ordering at a fast-food drive-through the doctor told me that I should go home and get my affairs in order, as I probably only had about three years to live, yet another traumatic event for me.

There was no comforting advice or hint of a possible cure on the horizon. No suggestions on how to improve my nutrition or any types of alternative treatments that might help. As I was leaving, he actually yawned and nonchalantly said to come back in a week. That was the first time I had laughed in days. It wasn't a happy laugh; it was an incredulous one. I knew if I continued to see that insensitive doctor I would end up dead within a year. I returned to our tour bus dazed but defiant. No matter what it took, I would find the doctor who would be my partner in my healing and who could give me what we all need most: hope. It took me some time, but I finally found "Dr. Right" for me, Dr. Bruce Bacon, who brought me through my worst fears of this insidious viral disease.

I faced a harsh foe in hepatitis C, one that took my singing career away and made even the least exertion daunting. But I fought back. Besides doing the medical treatment of a rigid course of interferon shots in my abdomen, I studied everything I could find on integrative types of healing. I learned about the brain and neuroscience along with the mind, body, and spirit connection, and psychoneurology.

I called on every current expert I could find. I pored over years of research and applied their knowledge and experience to my own disintegrating life. I practiced meditation, affirmations, and guided imagery of what my healthy body would look like. I went to biofeedback sessions, studied nutritional healing, had massages for my lymph system, saw a chiropractor, used aromatherapy, music, and pet therapy, incorporated mindfulness and spirituality, and read countless books and articles about how your belief impacts your immune system. When my health would allow, I attended seminars on natural modalities of healing and went to every lecture offered.

And I rested—a lot.

At one natural medicine seminar I listened to a keynote address given by Dr. Mona Lisa Schulz, a brilliant behavioral neuroscientist and neuropsychiatrist with a medical degree. She began practicing medical intuition almost thirty years ago and is one of the pioneers of studying, lecturing, and teaching about the relationships we have with health or illness. Her lecture resonated to my core. I had an intuitive feeling that she could play a big part in the hope that I was seeking.

In 1995, Dr. Bacon proclaimed me miraculously cured, entirely free of the hep C virus. I felt vibrant and full of life again. I shared my healing journey with everyone through a book and a speaking series. I was in demand as an inspirational speaker. I had a lot of placebo-based, double-blind clinical trials and good research to share. People wanted to hear my miraculous story, especially those in the medical field and those suffering with chronic illness, especially hepatitis C.

As I was descending into debilitating depression in 2012, I had a number of engagements as a keynote speaker, often at conventions of nurses, doctors, or medical practitioners, university professors and students, and community organizations. These engagements are usually booked a year ahead of the actual date. A few were scheduled for the spring of 2012. I knew I couldn't let people down. I'm extremely responsible.

I feel the most alive in front of groups of people. I absorb and reflect the energy of the audience and it brings me unbridled joy to know that I have information that can be shared and learned in an entertaining way.

In the past, I usually only required a bare outline of notes and a few PowerPoint slides and I was good for a forty-five-minute talk. I'd always been delighted to participate in a fast-paced question-and-answer period right after my speech. I was intrigued by the lives of others and I could always learn something from them, as well. But I could no longer imagine doing any of that, especially since the third prescribed antidepressant made me so anxious I constantly felt trapped in the confines of my own jumbled brain. I had no idea how I would pack a bag, prepare my talk, fly to the location, meet the coordinators, be social, and then give a worthwhile speech. I felt overwhelmed at the thought of it all.

When the time came to pack for these lectures that spring, I would stand at my closet door for long periods of time, not even able to pick out an appropriate outfit to wear. As soon as I would put something into the suitcase, I would have to check over and over again to make sure I had what I needed. I was scared I would show up with shoes that didn't match, or a skirt with no top. I packed and repacked my makeup bag, because I couldn't keep track of what I had already put in it. Once I had zipped up my suitcase, I would become extremely nervous that I had not packed pantyhose or the right bra and I would open it up and lay everything out all over again. This was totally unlike me. I'm always organized to the point of obsession. I had prided myself on the fact that I could probably pack a bag for two weeks in Europe within twenty minutes because I knew exactly where everything was. No longer.

I would get little sleep the night before the speaking engagement. I even traveled with a small one-cup coffeemaker, because I knew I'd be up at 4 a.m. preparing for the events of the day, long before room service could serve breakfast. I would pace the hotel room floor, rehearsing my talk over and over. By the time I was taken to the speaking venue, I would feel exhausted, but I wouldn't let on. I would laugh and chat with the other presenters as though nothing was wrong. When the host read my long introduction with all of the Judd career triumphs as well as my books and successful recovery from hepatitis C, the crowd would cheer and look up at me in anticipation of a humorous and uplifting report. They came to learn the secrets to my happy life. Little did they know that it had been six months since I had had a single moment of feeling happy or peaceful. If I wasn't in a zombie state lying on the couch, I had to keep myself from running screaming onto the freeway.

As I waited backstage, I would feel like bursting into tears and yelling at the top of my lungs. I wanted to be truthful and tell them that even though hepatitis C was hideous, it was minor compared to the misery I was going through with anxiety and depression. I wanted to shout out that I understood how people could get addicted to alcohol, heroin, and crack if they were in the emotional and physical pain I was suffering.

I wanted to confess that if someone took out a gun and killed me onstage he would be doing me a favor. But I didn't. The fans mean everything to me. I was there to regale them with stories and I was not going to disappoint. I gathered every ounce of strength I had, straightened my shoulders and did the twist to loosen up, adjusted my suit jacket, said a quick prayer, found the will to put a smile on my face, and strode out onstage. I never showed my mental anguish in public. By the end of the forty-five-minute talk I would feel like I had spent every bit of energy I had. I had not one more smile left in me.

After the third antidepressant proved to be ineffective, I told the psychiatrist that my anxiety was off-the-charts unbearable. He prescribed one of the four benzodiazepines, Klonopin, to take as needed. Klonopin slows down the brain function and blocks the receptors that signal anxiety and stress. Considering how I was feeling, it was something I started taking every four hours. It buffered the emotional and physical pain of my unbearable anxiety. It gave me the feeling that I could, once again, take a deep breath. The doctor also gave me prescription for Ativan, in hopes that my nighttime panic attacks would be less frequent. Over the course of the next year I also had prescriptions for two other benzodiazepines, Valium and Xanax, but Klonopin became the drug I depended on to get me through my most anxious days. And there were many of those.

In the past, I would have read extensively about every prescription, the success rate and the side effects. But one of the frustrating symptoms of my depression and anxiety is that I had no attention span at all. I would read one paragraph and then realize that I had no idea what I had just read, or I'd accidentally reread the same paragraph, over and over. I was desperate to find articles or research by someone who understood what I was going through.

I put myself in the hands of the professional. I took the prescribed antidepressants and Klonopin by day, and Ativan at night, even taking another when I would wake up at 3 a.m. This amount of antianxiety medicine left me groggy and emotionally flat.

In June 2012, I found out through *People* magazine that Wynonna had married her fiancé, Cactus, in her backyard. I wasn't invited and neither was Ashley. Wy was quoted in the press as saying that she wanted the wedding ceremony to be kept simple and small, only her and Cactus and their children from previous marriages. She also used the hands of a clock to describe the placement of our farms in this beautiful Tennessee countryside. She said that her home was at six o'clock and mine and Ashley's were at eleven and one. Her description could have been a metaphor of our relationships as mother and daughters. We operate from different points of view but each hand, though it moves independently, shares the same clock. We are three very strong-minded women, yet very impressionable, too, because of our emotional hearts, and time has never changed that. I was happy for Wy's marriage news, but sad at the same time. Because of my harsh upbringing, I will always long for the close family unity I didn't feel in my childhood.

It does satisfy me that my daughters think for themselves and are fiercely independent. But I'm still their mother. I worry when Ashley goes on her humanitarian missions, especially to countries that are politically volatile or have outbreaks of violence or disease. As I write this, Ashley is on an extensive trip to Jordan and Turkey working in refugee camps. But it's her passion, so I wouldn't try to change her, either.

Ashley and I are extremely close and have an unbreakable bond of understanding each other's needs. We share much in common: books, animals, outdoors, interesting people, community service, solitude, self-improvement, close friends, bluegrass music, state parks, and cooking. I appreciate that deeply. It's different with Wynonna because we spent almost all of our hours together from her birth to her preschool years, during my most turbulent times, all the way through intensive years of touring during her young adult years. Of course these are the years when most young people move away from their parents and live independently for the first time. We were constantly in the spotlight together, on and off stage. We had a public image to live up to and represent. It brought Wy and me close together in a mutual bond and it pushed us far apart because of the challenges of not having enough individuality. I think the OWN show being filmed during our Encore tour reminded us both of those feelings, because we were, once again, in the spotlight, on camera, on stage and off. The three of us had come through a lot together over the years and it hurt my heart that we couldn't all be together for happy times, like a wedding.

Chapter 6

The Future Isn't What It Used to Be

In July 2012, I thought I had hit an all-time low emotionally. I had concluded that I was of little value to anyone and had the lowest feelings of self-worth I had ever had my life.

Then, while changing into clean pajamas one evening, I found a large lump in my breast. It seemed like a sequel to a bad dream, one in which you wake up in fear, try to shake it off, and then fall right back to sleep and continue the same nightmare.

Larry set me up for a doctor appointment at Vanderbilt Breast Center. When the doctor told me that the mass seemed very worrisome and suggested an MRI, I wanted to leave immediately. The idea of being enclosed in a large metal tube for forty minutes was more than I could possibly bear. My anxiety started a steep ascent and I had a hard time catching my breath. Larry convinced me to go through with the test, pleading with me not to risk my physical health. Relying on Klonopin to keep me calm, I somehow made it through the test, with Larry speaking gently to me the entire time, reading scriptures from the Bible. The results of the MRI were inconclusive and so I was scheduled for a biopsy.

My nerves now felt like they had come through my skin and were exposed to the elements. No one, except Larry and Ashley, knew what I was going through. I didn't even call my group of "Ya-Ya" girlfriends.

I was admitted to the hospital, where under anesthesia I had a cluster of cells removed from my breast. In a couple of days, the doctor called with the good news that the results had come back negative but that I would have to keep an eye on the lump. Larry hugged me, smiling in relief. I was happy for him, but I could not feel much relief for myself.

Being away from Wynonna and having Ashley travel so often for her acting career or humanitarian work left me feeling desperately lonely for family. I still had great friends I could call, but during these days of extreme vulnerability, I longed for family. I craved a guaranteed stability, since I felt like I had none in my diseased brain. I wanted to bring my loved ones close and build a fortress around us all. I was deeply fearful that we would all drift apart. With my emotions feeling so out of control, I wanted to feel protected and surrounded by those who knew me best. I became even more terrified of being alone. I had to know where Larry was at all times. I didn't want him to leave my side.

If someone had told me that the fiercely independent Naomi Judd would become a nerve-racked, clingy wife, I would have laughed. Depression and anxiety had drastically changed my perspective on feeling safe and secure. I felt a pervading sense of danger or threat, like something worse might descend on me, even though I couldn't label it exactly. It was a heightened fear of the unknown future. Was the severity of my mental health a passing phase or would it forever be present, dooming my life to a misery I could never shake?

My fears of being alone brought up a long-buried sorrow, a heartbreaking memory of a time when another unknown factor first threatened, and then forever changed the stability of my family home.

On a warm Saturday morning when I was eighteen, I took my baby daughter over to my parents' house for a drop-in visit. My day-to-day life had changed drastically in the previous six months and I found myself yearning to be back with my parents and the familiarity of the house I grew up in, and away from the overbearing and constant critical attention of my perfectionist, controlling mother-in-law. Being at my childhood home made me terribly homesick.

As a daddy's girl, I was sad that we had grown distant with each other ever since the day he heard that I was pregnant. I thought it was all because of his disappointment in me, but that wasn't the only reason for his detached attitude. About thirty minutes after my arrival, he grabbed the keys to his truck and a small duffel bag. I chased after him to the front porch.

"Where are you going, Daddy?"

"Fishing," he said off-handedly, without looking back at me.

I knew he was fibbing because the bed of his pickup truck was completely empty. "Is your fishing stuff in the cab of the truck?" I asked.

He knew I was on to him. "I have to get my gear."

"Well, yeah!" I blurted out with a faltering conviction. "If you're really going fishing."

His shoulders drooped and he glanced at me dejectedly. "I'll be back home Sunday night, in plenty of time for work at the gas station on Monday."

I was trying really hard not to cry. I was terrified that he would never come back to us.

Mother joined me on the porch as Daddy drove off. "He's going to see her." She went back inside, to the kitchen, where she could always be found, for more than twenty years of their marriage, cooking, washing and ironing clothes, doing everything to take care of

Daddy and four children. My heart began to break. Sure, I had heard the rumors around town, but now my own mother was confirming that they were true.

A young woman who worked as a receptionist for Ashland Oil had begun dropping by Daddy's gas station on a regular basis. Her name was Cynthia, a semi-attractive girl who was only a couple of years older than me. In Ashland, Kentucky, in the 1960s, she was labeled "from the wrong side of the tracks." But she was smart enough to figure out a way to change sides quickly. She began flirting with Daddy whenever she could. For a few years, it appeared to be only a flirtation, but then everything took a turn in her favor. Daddy started spending overnights with her.

I wanted to dash into the kitchen and hold Mother, realizing that she had to be devastated. By the time I saw her, she was scrubbing the grease spots out of Daddy's work pants and acting like absolutely nothing was wrong.

Even if Mother could pretend everything was status quo, I couldn't. I had noticed that after Brian had died, my parents drifted apart. I was emotionally distraught that my father would cheat, but mostly I was appalled beyond measure that he would have an affair with this opportunistic young woman who could have been one of my schoolmates.

While I was living in Los Angeles, Daddy finally did leave home, never to return. He moved in with the demanding Cynthia and filed for a divorce. Soon after, he married her. I have no idea if he was in love; I suspect it was lust. True to our family pattern, we never spoke about his emotions or ours. However, I refused to accept her as a family member, this woman who appeared out of nowhere and had more influence over my father than my siblings and me or my mother.

Mother behaved like a vengeful fury once the reality of the situation sank in. For a number of years, she would not communicate with me at all. I didn't know why she shut down so completely against me, and she never explained. I believe it's because I didn't take sides and I wouldn't testify against Daddy at the divorce hearing. Because of her refusal to have anything to do with me, when I would visit Ashland, I would drive by our house and sit outside, watching her pace in front of the windows. I would bring a gift for her birthday or Christmas and leave it by her front door, run back to my car, and speed off. It broke my heart, knowing Mother was there alone.

Soon after Daddy died of kidney failure in 1984, I was tipped off by my cousin Chuck, whom Daddy thought of as another son, that Cynthia was attempting to keep the money and certificates of deposit Daddy had designated to go to my brother, sister, Chuck, and me. Now I knew for certain the exact type of greedy stepmother Cynthia really was. I took action and rushed to the bank the next day and marched into the manager's office with Chuck and my Daddy's lawyer in tow.

I lowered my voice and said, "I think you know why I'm here. A representative from the FDIC is right behind me, so I suggest you hand over the CDs within the next five minutes."

It worked. I didn't have a car at that time, so I used that money to buy one that belonged to Conway Twitty. Wy and I had been performing as the opening act for Conway's tour in 1984. He collected vintage automobiles of great style and offered to sell me his sublime turquoise '53 Cadillac. My daddy loved Caddys, so I used $10,000 of the money he left me to buy this extravagant car and drove it proudly.

But, a showpiece classic car was a shallow replacement for what I longed for most, a close and loving family. Looking back, fighting for the ten thousand dollars Daddy had left to me seemed an easy feat compared to winning unconditional acceptance or, at least, approval from either of my parents. I thought about how ironic it was that I had won the accolades of millions of fans, music critics, and song-writers from around the world, but was never able to believe that my own parents were happy for my success. Each time I had any expec-tation that they would be proud of me, my hopes were dashed.

A stinging heat flooded from my neck up to my face, the exact way it did the day I called my father from a pay phone to tell him that Wy and I had secured our very first recording deal after moving to Nashville. I had been living by my wits for years, and then working multiple shifts as a nurse to give Wy and me time to perform. On that golden day, after finally getting a chance to sing for RCA executives, we were told to wait in O'Charley's restaurant next to the studio while they deliberated whether we were talent they wanted to invest in.

I was ecstatic when the label men arrived with a handshake of congratulations and a promise of a recording contract. I grabbed a quarter, ran to the pay phone by the front door, and called my father. When he picked up the phone, I gushed out the fantastic news. I could hear Daddy exhale and I knew he was smoking one of his unfiltered Camel cigarettes.

"Isn't it exciting, Daddy? Our hard work is finally paying off. We have an RCA recording contract."

I could picture the exact setting my father was in more than three hundred miles away. He would be sitting in his red La-Z-Boy chair, with a TV tray by his side holding a Pepsi and a bowl of salted Planter's peanuts. His two little Westie dogs, Bonnie and Clyde, would be on his lap as he watched *Bonanza*. I heard him take a long drag on his cigarette again. Then he responded to my enthusiasm, without a single congratulatory word.

"You're not going to quit your nursing job, are you?"

"I don't know, Daddy." My elation turned to regret that I had called him. I wanted to slam the phone down.

After a couple of minutes of his telling me that it would be foolish to leave a stable job like nursing and that show business was not for "regular folk" like me, I could hear him set the dogs down on the floor and sit upright.

"Well, Cynthia has my dinner ready. Thanks for calling, honey."

My memory still holds that sting of rejection from the most important man in my life, ever.

There was only one thing that seemed to impress my father, out of all of my accomplishments. While watching one of his "regular folks" shows, he got to see Wy and me sing our number one song, "Mama, He's Crazy," on *Hee Haw*. To him that was the most impressive thing a simple girl from Ashland, Kentucky, could possibly do.

My bruised heart soon recovered from that phone call. Somewhere inside I flipped a switch from building a career to please my divorced parents to only doing it for Wy, Ashley, and me. As much as I could, I stayed true to that conviction, although I continually faced disappointment from my parents' inability to be happy for me, no matter what I did. I don't know why I had ever expected it, since neither of my parents ever had a moment of curiosity about what I wanted to do in the future or encouraged my educational pursuits or helped me to explore my options at all.

When I started my senior year of high school, I watched as my friends applied to various colleges. I was jealous that their parents would drive them to see the campuses and for interviews. My parents never once broached the subject of higher education; the word *college* was never spoken in our home, so I assumed it was something that I shouldn't even think about, though I dreamed of attending the

University of Kentucky. They lived meal to meal, chore to chore, and season to season.

I had broken away, jumped off the treadmill of dreary and monotonous daily life in the small town of Ashland, Kentucky. I had created a world for myself full of rich textures, new experiences, travel, and exciting ventures. But now that life had screeched to a halt.

As 2012 dragged on, I languished in my darkening misery on the kitchen couch. None of the antidepressants the psychiatrist had given me had improved my depression in the least. They actually caused my anxiety levels to break through to an even higher level. The psychiatrist tried me on a fourth antidepressant.

I would enthusiastically pop the next antidepressant, hoping, Maybe this one will work. I'll be free of this endless melancholy and get back my even disposition and optimistic outlook. After three weeks, which is about how long it takes for an antidepressant to have a full effect, I realized that the fourth was ineffectual, and if anything, I found facing a new day harder than ever.

My normally logical and commonsensical mind became impulsive and hair-trigger with thoughts that something had to happen or change "right now." After a week of dark days, both in the weather and my mood, I demanded that Larry sell our home and farm and that we move to California. To pacify me, Larry pretended to be searching for homes for sale in Del Mar, California. After endless misery, both day and night, a semblance of balance returned to my brain and I was frightened by my irrationality.

One day Larry encouraged me to go to the grocery store and pick out ingredients for dinner. It was the one trip out of the house that I could still be convinced to do. It was a way to be around people, but I didn't have to hold up a conversation or look nice. The bright lights and the colorful aisles gave my brain waves a temporary lift. As I stood in the produce aisle, I almost started to laugh. But it wasn't a chuckle of relief; it was the macabre laugh of a doomed person who realizes that there will be no escape.

Is this it? Is this all there is? I asked myself. This is now the highlight of my week? My whole life has now been reduced to squeezing melons in the produce aisle?

Larry asked me to try out a new church with him, thinking that a spiritual community would be a great support for me. I didn't want to go. I had not been to church in years, after attending every Sunday when we were in town.

We had always gone to the same Pentecostal church where Larry and I were married and Ashley was baptized. Wynonna had married her first husband there. I thought it would be the church I attended for the rest of my life, until one Sunday the pastor decided to warn the congregation about the sinfulness and degradation of homosexuality. He advised the congregation that our children needed to be protected from gay people. I was stunned. Many of the people I've worked with over the years have been gay, both men and women. Far from needing to "protect ourselves" from gay people, I've always found it to be quite the opposite. My gay coworkers and friends have always protected me, taken care of me professionally, and stood up for me over the years. A number of my fans are gay. They have been loyal and loving for three decades and seeing their faces in the audience at my concerts with Wynonna has always made me feel a deep gratitude. The offensive words of the pastor had barely traveled to the back of the sanctuary before I was on my feet to leave, never to set foot in my home church again.

I thought about all of the hardships I had overcome in my life: being sexually abused as a child, losing my brother to cancer, teenage pregnancy, betrayal and abandonment by the birth father, my divorce, single motherhood, poverty, being on welfare following my divorce, sleeping on a deloused mattress from Goodwill, having to escape Los Angeles because of an ex-con stalker who raped and beat me, then living in a fishing cabin with no heat while putting myself through nursing school and working two other jobs, and overcoming a life-threatening disease, hepatitis C. Through it all, I had prayed.

I was done praying. Why would a loving God let me sink so low now? Why would he let the disease in my brain become so unpredictable and my thoughts so dark? I felt that God was a phony and had abandoned me to this hideous mental illness, and I was mad as hell at him. My faith withered away. I went into spiritual exile.

I told Larry that I couldn't go to any church with him. Larry would hold me in his arms, but he was running out of words to comfort me.

One gloomy November morning, sitting on the edge of the bed, I was thinking about being onstage and how much joy I felt at the end of each concert. I wanted everyone in the audience to leave feeling really good, too. Wy and I would sing the Judds' most widely known hit, "Love Can Build a Bridge." It's a song I wrote for our millions of fans the year I became ill with hepatitis C. It won a Grammy for Best Country Song. During my acceptance speech at the awards show I joked, "I don't deserve this, but I have hep C and I don't deserve that, either."

"Love Can Build a Bridge" is an anthem of strength and recovery. Some of the lyrics: "I would swim out to save you, in your sea of broken dreams. When all your hopes are sinkin', let me show you what love means."

Here I was drowning, but I couldn't save myself. I didn't know where the hopelessness came from, so I could only think of one way to get rid of it. Love can build a bridge, but in my despair I was considering other ways that a bridge could end my pain.

Chapter 7

Do Your Genes Fit?

knew exactly how I was going to carry out my suicide. I wouldn't park at one end of the bridge, where people might stop me or question what I was doing. I would drive my car to the very center, the highest point, and in one swift motion open the car door and climb over the railing. I'd keep my focus on the beauty of the surrounding countryside, spread my arms out, and step off. After the 155-foot drop to State Route 96 below, it would all be over, now and forever. I would be out of this relentless torment.

The Natchez Trace Parkway Bridge was completed in 1994. It's thirteen miles from my house and was built as one of the last sections of the Natchez Trace Parkway. There's a palpable sense of history along the Natchez Trace: Native American ceremonial mounds, Civil War battlefields, Victorian homes, forests, and farmlands, a record of more than two hundred years of history. The Natchez Trace Bridge is one of only two post-tensioned arch bridges in the world. Perhaps it could provide a post-tension solution for me.

Despite winning awards for design and originality, the Natchez Trace Bridge holds another distinction. There has been at least one suicide per year from the bridge since its completion. Ironically, the sheriff of our town had recently approached me about helping him acquire the funds to add safety nets on both sides of the bridge to save any poor soul who decided to commit suicide by jumping. I told him, "I'll get back to you on that one."

I have been a personal friend for more than twenty-five years of Dr. Francis Collins, who was the director of the National Human Genome Research Institute. We met when we were both being inducted into the Academy of Achievement, a nonprofit that honors notable people for student educational purposes. He was being honored in the Science and Exploration category and I was for the Arts and as a Social Advocate. He's an introspective and brilliant physician and genetic scientist who has spent much of his professional life decoding human DNA. His work has given us the ability to "read our own instruction book." His discoveries have helped develop a method of screening the human gene for diseases. One of his main interests is the way inheritance from our ancestors influences disease.

Francis and Diane, his lovely wife, who is a genetics counselor, came to vacation for a week at our farm. Going through years of recovery from hepatitis C gave me a ravenous appetite to listen and learn from the experts, wherever and whenever I can find them. Luckily for me, I had the chance to host Dr. Collins at my own kitchen table, where he answered my questions and coached me as we ate chicken and dumplings.

Now, in my darkened state of mind, I heard echoes of a tantalizing fact I had learned from Dr. Collins. He explained to me that mental illness is often a family disease. If a parent has depression or anxiety, then their child has about a 50 percent chance of having it. When both parents have a mental illness, the child's chances of having one as well goes up to 75 percent. The Centre for Addiction and Mental Health, in Toronto, had determined that about 90 percent of people with suicidal thoughts have at least one mental health disorder. I had also read that studies from as recently as 2011 were uncovering a strong genetic biomarker in families with suicidal tendencies.

This was one of those circumstances where "ignorance is bliss." The statistics of inherited mental illness terrified me. Though I've always considered myself the one who broke the mold of what a determined girl from Ashland, Kentucky, could do with her future, there was no denying that my family history on both sides was like the variety pack of mental illness. More than that, every generation in my family had a suicide that changed the family dynamics forever. Would I be another statistic? Other families pass down treasured heirlooms or historical artifacts. My family shuffled a horrendous tendency to suicidal ideation onto subsequent generations, starting with my great-great-grandfather David Oliver.

My mother's grandfather, David was a stonemason in Portsmouth, Ohio. He cheated on his young wife, Tilly, mercilessly; after years of dealing with his infidelity she fled to her parents' home in Portsmouth. David's unpredictable and destructive behavior would later be diagnosed as mental illness, but at the time he was labeled as an unpredictable drunk. In a fit of rage and revenge against Tilly, David, inside the house, sealed the doors and windows of his home and turned on the gas. But he wasn't alone. Their two innocent little sons, Howard and Norman, ages seven and five, were in the house with him. He sat them on the couch and then proceeded to make a rope noose and throw it over a beam across the ceiling. David stood on a chair, pulled the noose over his head, and kicked the chair out from under him. The little boys were already suffering the effects of asphyxiation from the wide-open gas pipe. Terrified and starting to feel sick, the older son, seven-year-old Howard, knew that they, too, would soon die.

Howard crawled to the window at the end of the room. He opened the window and fresh air poured into the room. He crawled out onto the flat roof, pulling his five-year-old brother, Norman, to safety. Peering back over the windowsill, little Howard slowly realized his own father was trying to murder them while committing suicide. No one knows why Tilly would leave her children's fates in the hands of a man with such an unstable mental condition, but history would reveal a long line of relatives who passed on a narcissistic personality disorder. She didn't even return for her sons following their father's suicide. The boys had to go through a court system, until eventually one of Tilly's relatives rescued them from an orphanage.

Scientists in a 2007 study reported in the *International Journal of Neuropsychopharmacology* found a specific gene implicated in the development of narcissistic personality disorder and which has a very high rate of heritability. Neither of the boys ever fully recovered emotionally from this unimaginable shock, although it seemed to affect the younger boy, Norman, more.

I grew up around him and observed that he was very withdrawn and rarely spoke after that. Throughout his life, his physical stance was as stiff as that of a vintage cigar store Indian. There were no psychological services available in those days, especially out in the country, but there certainly was a lot of gossip. Word spread fast and the boys had to face the daily whispers of their classmates and the townspeople.

The older boy, redheaded and quiet Howard, was to become my mother's dad, my grandfather. When my mother, Polly, was only eleven years old, Howard, who had survived his father's suicide–double murder attempt, was found dead in his bathroom, shot in the head.

No one explained to young Polly what had happened to her father. Apparently it didn't matter to her mother, Edie Mae, that her husband had seemingly committed suicide, leaving her with three small children. The coroner labeled Howard's death a suicide, but Edie Mae's own mother, my great-grandmother Cora Lee, knew that her daughter had murdered her husband.

Edie Mae left town soon after with her secret lover, Jerry, unceremoniously dumping her three children off at Cora Lee's house. She only returned to live with her mother, once again, after Jerry died of an accidental electrocution. Edie Mae never took responsibility for her three children. She was a textbook example of an extreme narcissist, and a possible psychopath.

My great-grandma Cora Lee ran a popular diner on Main Street in Ashland, called the Hamburger Inn, which took up most of her time. My orphaned teenage mother was left to raise her two siblings, even as she began to work at the restaurant as free child labor. It sure made sense to me that my mother never, ever referred to Edie Mae as "Mom" or "Mother."

Edie Mae, instead of behaving like a mother, was a silly, flirtatious, and flippant loudmouth. She had gaudy fire-orange hair and wore way too much makeup as she paraded through town, hoping to meet a man for drinks at the VFW. She spent money wildly on herself and her friends, leaving her children to scrape together the necessities as best they could. My mother was the one who made sure her two siblings, Norman and Martha Lee, were clean and fed and kept up with their schoolwork. Mother signed her siblings' report cards and helped them get primped up for any school dances.

I was frightened of Edie Mae as a small child. One afternoon, during an unwelcome visit, she told me to paint her fingernails, as she leaned toward my face with her brittle, processed hair nearly in my eyes and her stale alcohol breath wafting into my nose. My stomach did a flip-flop in fear of having to spend any time with her, so I came up with an excuse that I had left something important outside. I flew out the door and down the sidewalk and rounded the corner out of Edie Mae's sight. I couldn't believe this weird woman was my grandmother. But she really wasn't. She never hugged me or acted as if she cared about my existence. Why would she care about her granddaughter when she was such a self-absorbed narcissist that she never cared about what happened to her own children?

In a rare moment when Mother was open to talking about her childhood, I asked her if she ever loved Edie Mae. She dismissed the question with a flick of her wrist and a disgusted sigh, saying, "It's hard to have love for someone who never pays any attention to you."

Edie Mae spent her last years in an abysmal county nursing home for the destitute. My mother went to see her a couple of times before she passed away. I always wanted to ask Mom if she had been aware her mother had murdered her father. Edie Mae never had any remorse for killing her husband, Howard, for abandoning her children, or for her extravagant waste of the family's minimal resources. Her only request, fitting the true narcissistic template, was to demand that my mother take her to live in her home. Fat chance!

The only personal belonging that Mother has from her mother is an ornate clasp, a buckle that was on the belt of a luxurious long black velvet coat that Edie Mae wore on special occasions. I've watched as my mother has held the clasp in her hands, turning it over and over as if she might find the secret code to forgiving her selfish mother, or as if it might have some magical attributes that could revise heartache and history. I find it oddly symbolic that the one memento she kept is a clasp, something meant to hold two separate things together.

My mother is a survivor. In her early life, she endured more psychological damage than most people endure in a lifetime. She has been an example to me in that respect. She lived in a crowded, cigarette-smoke-filled house, where the curtains were always drawn. She shared a small bedroom with her siblings, because Cora Lee's other five oddball adult children, my mom's aunt and uncles, all had mental and addiction problems and had either never left home or had returned after a brief but unsuccessful foray out in the real world. None of them seemed capable of making decisions and all seemed lost without their mother, Cora Lee, running their lives and having them help her with the restaurant.

When my father first met my mother, while eating lunch at the Hamburger Inn, and showed interest in her, Mother felt a flicker of hope that this hardworking young man could rescue her. My vulnerable fifteen-year-old mom jumped at her chance to escape her harsh childhood and married this eighteen-year-old man. When she was eighteen, she gave birth to me. She became a full-time housewife to whom the meager life my father carved out for her felt like a step up from the lifestyle she had endured for her first fifteen years of life.

My daddy was a nice enough looking young man who put in twelve to fourteen hour days at his gas station six days a week. He was straightforward, honest as the day is long, and undemonstrative. Every day one of us would take him a brown-bag lunch Mother had made. When he came home he wanted his supper. She always had it ready for him. Mother was a fabulous cook from her years of experience in the restaurant. We never lacked for a meal of comfort food, like fried chicken, mashed potatoes, green beans, and homemade fudge for dessert.

The neighborhood kids would always want to visit, because they knew my mother would have a plate of snickerdoodle cookies or a pie or two set out on the counter.

I think it was the enthusiasm we all showed for her food that made Mother feel appreciated. It's one time when I saw her happy and expressive, so I always tried to make sure I brought my friends into the house, even though I would have to run around gathering up and throwing all of the clutter left around the living room into a clothes hamper or shove it under the couch to hide it. She may have been a great cook but she rarely stepped outside the kitchen to see if the rest of the house was in order.

Even though our kitchen was often bustling with neighbor kids, I never once saw my parents ask any adults over. We never had any company, except for a few relatives, only once or twice a year. Daddy coached Little League games for my brothers, and Mother would bake for the PTA sale, but neither one had any hobbies. It appeared my parents didn't need the connection, happiness, or comfort of having friends. They didn't express the slightest amount of affection toward each other. They never hugged or kissed in front of me or even held hands. There was never any overt display of affection in our home at all. I don't remember ever getting a congratulatory pat on the back for a job well done.

My mom would cook, bake, and do laundry, watch after us, and keep my father in clean work clothes. He would work until seven, come home, scarf down his plate of food, and retire to his red recliner to watch boxing or some western or gangster movie, leaving Mother and me to clean up the dishes. I never once saw my dad bring her a gift or flowers, or even give her a card on her birthday, yet she never complained. Her only friends were Kitty, a woman whom she grew up with and who stood as the witness at her wedding to my father, and my aunt Roberta, who had an equally hard life married to my uncle Norman, an alcoholic who eventually abandoned his family of three and began to live as a gay man.

I don't know if my parents ever said the words "I love you" to each other. I certainly never heard it. But I do know that Mother was a dedicated martyr to Daddy. When, after twenty-five years of marriage, Daddy decided to walk out on us and move in with Cynthia, his twenty-three-year-old mistress, the humiliation, gossip, and the betrayal left Mother devastated. I observed her gradually becoming judgmental, bitter, and negative to the bone and I found out that she was throwing and smashing dishes.

I was living in Hollywood, with Michael and Wynonna, and Ashley was still an infant, when the phone rang in the middle of the afternoon. It was Daddy. I knew something was wrong, because he never called me. I always had to check in on him, and after he had plans to marry Cynthia, I rarely had the urge to call him. It was as if Daddy had become a different person, one who had left his past behind, as if Mother and we children had never existed.

"Your mother was found unconscious in her car," Daddy sputtered, plunging ahead with the awful news, giving me no time to prepare. "She overdosed on pills. She's in the ICU."

I couldn't picture Mother doing this. She had come to Hollywood when Ashley was born, to meet her new granddaughter and help out with Wynonna, who was still a rambunctious toddler. It was obvious then that Mother was still very angry with Daddy, but I didn't see it as hopelessness, only bitterness. Apparently the cold, hard reality of her situation had now settled in for good. She had to face the fact that Daddy was not coming back to her. She was trapped in a mire of embarrassing rejection and humiliation as a divorced woman in a town where divorce wasn't common and most women didn't work outside the home.

A police officer had come upon her car, parked on an isolated dead-end country road that backed up to a field behind Cynthia's apartment building. This was a "lover's lane" where teenagers would play hooky from school and smoke pot or make out. The officer expected to see a couple of delinquent teenage boys hiding out in the car instead of a pretty auburn-haired housewife, slumped sideways on the seat, whose lips and forearms were now a pale shade of grayish-blue from lack of oxygen, an empty bottle of prescription Valium on the seat next to her. The officer alerted an ambulance and Mother was taken to King's Daughters' Hospital emergency room, where they managed to save her life by pumping her stomach repeatedly. She was most likely minutes from death when the officer found her.

Even though I had been relieved to move across the country and escape the dreariness of Ashland and the demands of Michael's parents, to sunny, hip, fast-paced Hollywood, I was now panicked at the thought of Mother dying with me so far away.

Would our relationship end this way, without any expression of love between us? We were not only emotionally distant from each other, but also 2,300 miles apart.

"What will happen to her, Daddy?" I asked, my voice shaking.

"I bought you an airplane ticket," Daddy explained. "Bring the girls with you. The Ciminellas will have to keep them at their house, because I don't know how long you will have to stay."

About twenty-four hours later, I was at her bedside in the intensive care unit. Although her eyes were open and I was sure she recognized me, she was fairly unresponsive. For the first day, I sat by her bed, just trying to think of anything to offer to keep her alert and responsive.

The second day, she began to speak. After the third day it was obvious that her brain had survived the drug overdose and oxygen deprivation. Her one request was for me to bring in food so she didn't have to eat a hospital kitchen dinner. The doctors released Mother from the hospital without a single suggestion that she seek mental health help. They sent her home without any psychological follow-up or therapy. I felt stunned and dismayed. After all she had been through, beginning in childhood, she never went through counseling. When I tried to talk to her about the overdose, she acted as if it was all a big misunderstanding and wasn't really a suicide attempt at all.

I stayed on with her for another week, while she drank endless cups of coffee at our kitchen table and spoke derisively about Daddy living with his mistress and the way she was now forever shamed in front of the whole community. I could tell my mother was terrified at the prospect of being alone and losing all she had, which, at this point, was our family home.

"This is what I get for working like a dog," she lamented. "And being a stay-at-home mom." She slapped her palms down on the table like an exclamation point.

She ignored my attempts at sympathy and only wanted to deplore her chances of getting by on her own, with no income, since she had never worked other than as a homemaker after she married Daddy. The one thing my mother always did extremely well was cook, so I told her that it wouldn't be difficult to find a job. Living on the Ohio River, there were cargo riverboats always looking for a cook to feed the many men who worked on board for weeks at a time. On my suggestion, she went to meet with a river pilot, who hired her on the spot. The weathered, lonely riverboat captain fell for my unaffectionate and bitter mother and they married a few years later despite the fact that he couldn't hold an intelligent discussion about anything except riverboats. Still, the job gave Mother a feeling of accomplishment and she continued to work on the river until her retirement.

Now I contemplated how my leap from the bridge would leave absolutely no chance that Ashley or Wy would sit by my bedside in a hospital ICU. I could desperately use the emotional support and advice of a loving mother, but I didn't even think about calling her. I had never known her to reciprocate any of my attempts to be supportive and loving toward her. Why would that start now?

In any case, I was certain that the inheritance of mental illness and suicide in my family had been passed to me. The bridge seemed to be my final stop, my preordained destiny.

The next evening, my grandson Elijah came to the house with his girlfriend, Haley, to have our usual Thursday night dinner with Larry, Ashley, and me. He is a handsome, tough-looking, yet tender-hearted young man who has always been very close to me and whom I adore.

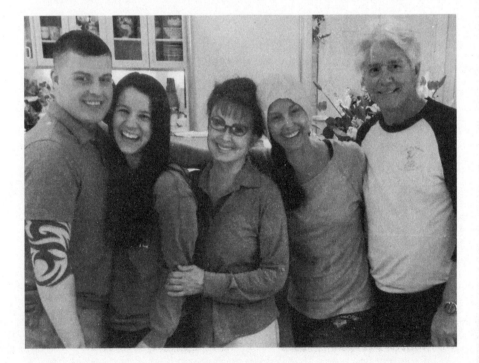

As we sat at the dinner table, Elijah relayed the details of how he had heard about a police officer who had to respond to a suicide from the Natchez Trace Bridge the previous night. Even though the person who had jumped was a stranger, Elijah disclosed how upset it made him feel to think of finding someone's body after they leapt from that bridge. I had to excuse myself and leave the table. I went into the bathroom to weep. The thought of my beloved grandson being the person who could possibly have to identify my mangled body was more than I could bear.

I felt such a deep shame about not being able to shake off this increasingly dark and immobilizing depression. The only thing sparing me from suicide was the effect it would have on those I loved, and all of the people who thought of me as a hope seller, but the odds were beginning to weigh against them. The disease in my brain was as persistent as the hepatitis C virus had been in my liver. I began to convince myself that I was a waste of breath and life. After our company left that night, I called Dr. Mona Lisa Schulz, even though it was already past midnight in Maine, where she lives.

"Hello," she answered, obviously woken from a deep sleep.

I sat silently, for what seemed like a full minute. In my head, I was making a decision: Would I reach out and ask my friend to save me, or should I hang up right now and find a way to end my life quickly?

"Hello. Who is this? Naomi?" She sounded groggy and I could hear her bedside lamp click on.

Then I heard a flat, unemotional, and unfamiliar voice say, "Can you help me? I'm very, very sick."

Chapter 8
Paging Doctor Schulz

Without asking many questions, my dear friend of two decades, Dr. Mona Lisa, as I call her, caught a plane from Maine to be by my side. I'm sure Larry was now less worried, knowing she was on her way. He had witnessed me slipping downhill for more than a year now and was hoping Dr. Mona Lisa could help me because not only is she a PhD neuroscientist and an MD; she's also a psychiatrist.

At any other time, I would have been overjoyed that my long-time friend was coming to our farm, but I had sunk so low and my emotions were so flat I couldn't feel anything at all: no happiness, no optimism, no anticipation of better days.

I did my best to explain my ineffectual experience with my Nashville psychiatrist and I listed for her the many antidepressants he had put me on during the past year, one after another. Being a person who is a medical intuitive, using her intuition to describe all of the factors, both emotional and physical, that are contributing to an individual's health problems, as well as a physician who has been formally educated in the consequences of mistreated depression, Dr. Mona Lisa was very concerned.

Using her vast resources of psychiatry reference books written by top specialists, Dr. Mona Lisa had researched the medications I told her I had been prescribed. She sat with me and explained the uses and side effects of every single antidepressant and antianxiety medication I had been on. By the end of 2012 and into the first few months of 2013, I had gone through serial courses of Prozac, Celexa, Zoloft, Lexapro, Wellbutrin, Paxil, Abilify, and Luvox. For my panic disorder, I had taken all four of the benzodiazepines: Xanax, Ativan, Valium, and Klonopin, one right after another. Nothing was working.

Dr. Mona Lisa explained that with an SSRI, you have to gradually cease taking one over three to seven days and then wait three to fourteen days before trying another. I was currently on three simultaneously. It is also well known among competent psychiatrists that an antidepressant won't work until the patient's anxiety disorder is under control, because one of the side effects of some antidepressants is anxiety. As she looked up each of the drugs I had been prescribed, she shook her head in disbelief.

As Dr. Mona Lisa read the side effects, I could check almost every one: severe insomnia, weight gain of twenty pounds, hair loss, memory loss, fatigue, blurred vision, constipation, and loss of libido. The side effect that really caught my ear was "hostility events." The only emotions I felt anymore were despair and anger. The Naomi my dear friend Dr. Lisa knew, the woman who loved humor, humanity, physics, learning about genetics, and hearing about the latest findings in neuroscience and healing techniques, was now a woman who would probably be kicked off an airplane for her foul mouth.

My husband, Larry, would cringe at my crude language as he watched me spiral down day by day. The genteel lady who used to walk out of movies that were too risqué or used foul language now yelled obscenities at the least little provocation. I'd make fun of people I didn't even know. I'd make disparaging remarks about someone taking my parking space and then feel mortified I had expressed those thoughts out loud. I couldn't explain why. It was almost as if a rebellious and infuriated teenager had taken over my mind. This gave me one more reason to stay at home, in familiar company. The rage that was right under the surface at any given moment was a complete 180 from who I had always been: happy, thoughtful of others, and tolerant.

Dr. Mona Lisa left Franklin to return to her practice in Maine, vowing to be there for me, and making me promise that I would keep her updated on my treatments. She advised me to look into finding a different psychiatrist locally. What I learned from Dr. Mona Lisa's well-educated perspective is that my depression and anxiety was a very delicate balancing act to treat, one that was so complicated it might take some time to resolve. A structured intense therapy would help with the psychological and social aspects of depression, but the biological changes were beyond my control.

Depression has a profound affect on the neurotransmitters. Only in recent years have there been intensive studies of the biology of depression, but what researchers already know is that a reduction in dopamine and serotonin, the "happy chemical" in your brain, and norepinephrine, a hormone released by the sympathetic nervous system, which controls our "fight or flight" response, is common with depression. Depression and anxiety go hand in hand with high levels of stress hormones, which can have a variety of negative effects on a person's biology, especially the adrenal glands. Even though none of this was good news, I was at least grateful to have some information. I knew there had to be some logical reason I was finding myself in such a dark and scary place.

I was reminded of the healing aspect of having a doctor who can take the time to listen first, give helpful information, and have a respectful dialogue with the patient. Dr. Mona Lisa told me that most doctors listen to their patients only for an average of nineteen seconds before interrupting and diagnosing. As an RN, I had observed this, too. If your doctor doesn't have time to listen to you, then you are not being served; you're being serviced, like a car that gets another oil change and is sent out the door. No mechanic cares about a car's feelings. They just fix what they think needs to be fixed. That shouldn't be true of your doctor. Ever.

Before the depression had descended on me in full, I had signed on to play the character role of Rita in a Hallmark Christmas movie *Window Wonderland,* which was to be shot in Vancouver in early 2013. I had not given it much thought because I was certain that I would be back to feeling like myself long before a full year and three months had gone by. But, the truth is, I was feeling worse than ever. I've never been one to neglect a commitment, even though I was concerned about being able to keep up mentally and physically on the movie set. Airline tickets were arranged and I packed for my acting job. Usually I would be thrilled to be spending time on a movie set, but I worried that my professional peers would be able to see that I was struggling with major depression and anxiety.

Each day I arrived on the set with my lines learned and a big smile on my face. I would spend an hour or two with the makeup and hair crew as they got me ready to be on camera. They would hug me and tell me jokes and stories about their lives and by the time my makeup was on, I would feel uplifted enough to get through the rigorous day. It reminded me of how crucial social and physical contact is to our sense of well-being. I don't think they had any idea how much I counted on their supportive chats and lighthearted humor to jump-start my day. I began to feel a confidence and a sense of belonging.

There was an unexpected upswing to my state of mind, which I noticed about three days into the filming schedule. I had something to look forward to, a distraction that gave my tumultuous mind a reprieve from unbearable depression and loneliness. I definitely wasn't back to feeling like myself, but luckily for me I didn't have to play myself. Being able to step into a role and become a woman named Rita for those three weeks was a calming respite. Pretending to have a different life, even for a day, was like being in the still eye of the emotional hurricane that was ravaging my mind. While I was in character, I could let go of Naomi and all the issues that came along with being me. I would flip a switch and not think about anything except the fun part I was playing.

At night, in my hotel room, I would think about the scenes we had shot that day and review my lines for the next day. Then I would go to sleep early. It was interesting to observe that I slept peacefully all night with no panic attacks. Being on location for filming, alongside an enthusiastic cast and crew and the "family vibe" on a set, gave me the same comforting, secure feeling as being on tour.

However, like a tour, filming a movie also comes to an end. It was a rude awakening to go back to having no character to escape into every day. Once again, on the plane ride home, I found myself fighting back the tears. I scolded myself with harsh thoughts: Naomi Judd, what is so wrong with your everyday life that you dread going home? The only answer I could come up with is that there was nothing wrong with my very fortunate world, there was only something wrong with my brain.

I was lost to myself. I had re-created and reinvented myself from the time I left Ashland at age eighteen. I had figured out who and what I needed to become to survive. I had become very good at doing that. I didn't stop to look back, because I didn't have time to do so. Stopping would have meant starving, or being put out on the street. I had to take care of my two daughters and myself. Whatever hurt me, including most of my childhood, was squashed down under the surface, locked away where it couldn't damage my chances of survival. But now, with nothing but time on my hands, my past trauma was back with an agenda.

The Naomi Ellen Judd who was emerging from the background of a life full of disappointments and tragedies was determined to take center stage and speak her mind. Naomi Judd the superstar would have to settle for a back-row seat in the audience. But I wasn't ready to switch places. The stubborn optimism that had carried me through thick and thin didn't want to listen to the frightened and abandoned young girl I had long left behind. I had worked too hard to build a world for myself. All I knew was that I had to find a permanent solution to get back to a healthy frame of mind, ignoring the fact that my world was still spinning out of my control.

Not only was I trying to contain a brewing rage from my childhood and young adult years, which I had never resolved. I also had yet to come to terms with my current life and the fears I had about my ongoing lack of connection with Wynonna. I felt that our relationship was getting more and more distant by the day. She was unaware of my struggles with depression and continued to focus on her new marriage and the formation of her new band and a huge remodeling project on her house. How could she have any idea of what I was going through, since I wasn't telling her? When we had toured together, we were always in sync in terms of knowing the other's emotions, the good ones as well as those of sorrow, frustration, and worry. I thought that our lifelong symbiotic relationship would override any differences we had at the end of the Encore tour. Why wouldn't she intuitively know that I was spiraling downward emotionally and reach out to me? As the months went by, I grew increasingly lonely for a connection with her. No one else could fill that space for me. But I was caught between an unresolvable rock and a hard place. As her mother, I didn't want to appear weak and vulnerable, but I still wanted my daughter's emotional support. There had been a time when we could practically read each other's minds; not so much now.

Once I returned home from filming the Hallmark movie, I struggled to stay afloat, like a bug that has fallen into a bucket of rainwater. But like the bug in the pail, I just treaded water, going around and around in circles, not getting anywhere, and sensing that I would soon drown in my own depression.

I found myself unmotivated to get dressed or even prepare a meal. Larry would come and sit on the kitchen couch next to me and try to talk me into going out for dinner or a movie, but I didn't have any interest in leaving the house.

My dog, Maudie, who is about as close to human as a canine can get, would gaze at me with her sympathetic deep brown eyes and then rest her chin on the couch cushion near my face. She can read my mind and can tell what I want her to do without me saying a word. She has always been protective of me, but she clearly felt uneasy about what was going on. I was becoming a stranger to her. I believe that dogs can recognize human suffering and I know that is true for Maudie. I rescued her as a scrubby, red-coated, mutt puppy in a large litter, but throughout these years of depression she has returned that favor a million times. She became my "therapy dog." She loves me unconditionally. Maudie rescued me on many dark days by staying nearby, like a four-legged guardian angel.

Everything started to bother me now that I was home, and, once again, an inner rage began to surface in ways that felt unpredictable and scary. Each new day was a repeat of the previous one, with me smoldering in frustration that there was nothing I could do to lift this baneful depression. I would feel another bout of strong anger coming on, but I didn't have an outlet for it. Often I would go up into the bedroom, shut the door, and punch pillows.

One afternoon, I had so much restless despair about my situation, I could no longer languish on the couch. It was gray and dull outside and I felt closed in and forgotten. Larry had gone into his home office to work, leaving me to myself. I wanted to do something dramatic, to shake myself up.

My body took action, getting me off the couch and upstairs. I decided to take Larry's substantial collection of guns for a test drive. I think my brain was so overloaded with overlapping prescriptions of antidepressants, now working counterproductively. Instead of bringing me a level of calm from the storm, they brought on a rage like I had never felt before. I had to let it out somewhere and somehow. I opened the safe and packed a duffel bag with the guns and ammunition, including the guns with clips. Then I slung it over my shoulder, snuck out the back door, and walked into our valley. My feet slid precariously beneath me on the damp earth and mud began to cake around the edges of my slippers. I almost laughed out loud thinking about what I must have looked like: a woman in her silk pajamas and an orange hunting cap, treading awkwardly down a slippery grass slope, with a bag of loaded firearms.

A rotted tree had become uprooted during the winter and had fallen over, resting heavy against a nearby living tree. It seemed to represent how I felt about myself: no longer grounded in her true self and slowly dying, rotting from the inside out.

I set the duffel bag on the ground and took out a Ruger 357. I fired all six of the bullets into the dead tree. The sound of the gun discharging carried me out of my own thoughts and made my heartbeat quicken. The noise made my brain feel like it was snapping awake and I felt truly alert for the first time in a year. When the first gun was out of ammunition, I took another out of the bag and repeated the process. The dead tree shook with the force of the bullets, but never fell to the ground. The branches of the live tree held it upright despite the barrage that should have toppled it. By the time I got to the fourth gun, Larry came racing over the crest of the valley. We allow hunters on our property at certain times of the year, but he suddenly realized that the noise on our property was not coming from a regular hunter. He took the gun slowly from my hands and gently led me back up to the house. We walked in silence. I think he knew that words weren't necessary. He only held his arm around my waist, like the strong tree, keeping me from collapsing to the ground.

Larry decided, without consulting me, to hide all the guns following this incident. What he didn't know was that, days before, I had put a small Ruger in the toe of a boot in my closet. I wanted to have options when I was certain I couldn't go on one more day. I had the bridge, the gun, and enough pills stockpiled to get out of pain for good. I still thought about it every single day.

When Larry and I went to bed that night, I warned him that I didn't know how much lower I could possibly go and that I was sorry and felt so guilty for putting him through this miserable time. He had unselfishly stayed by my side supporting me through my three years of recovering from hepatitis C.

He told me that helping me through that physical illness was easier than seeing my mental and emotional pain. He confided that he didn't feel as powerless then, because we had the diagnosis and we could take actual steps to help heal my ailing liver. The brain is a different story, the most mysterious part of the body. I know we both felt that finding an antidepressant that would finally help me was the only hope.

In April 2013, Larry sat on the edge of our bed and delivered the news that our neighbor and my country music hero George Jones had died. To me George was the true king of country music. When I was a starving nursing student in Marin County, California, I saved my change in the corner of my top dresser drawer. When I read in the paper that George Jones was performing nearby, I dug out the change to buy tickets for Wynonna and me. We sat in awe of this country music icon, listening to his distinctive voice glide from tenor to baritone and back. No one could sing of heartbreak and hardships like George. To this day, I think his talent surpasses any male country singer who ever lived. He would never have agreed because he was extremely humble.

Years after attending that concert, following an awards show, when the Judds were new to the country music scene, he invited me to visit him on his tour bus. Here was this rather crotchety and gruff man who was cuddling a tiny, pure white Maltese puppy that he wanted to show off. He had named her Star. Seeing him with that little dog, I gained an even deeper admiration for George and we became friends.

He didn't give two hoots about the accolades or awards. His only passion was to sing. He was certainly not an easy person to be around, but he was an authentic one. The news of his death devastated me. I felt as if any interest I had in country music might go to the grave with George.

I pulled the covers up and turned over. I didn't get out of bed that day. I didn't eat a single thing and I drank very little water. I didn't get out of bed the next day, either. Or, for the next five days. I didn't bathe, brush my teeth, or change my pajamas. I had no idea if it was day or night or how many days had passed. Larry tried to encourage me often to eat something, to sit up and watch a TV show. I waved him away, refusing the protein smoothies he brought to my bedside.

Larry told me I had been asked to speak at George's memorial service. That was impossible. I was slowly becoming incoherent. I wanted to fall asleep and never wake up again. At one point, I started to hallucinate, seeing flashes of painfully bright light or dark figures approaching from my peripheral vision. I saw my brother, Brian, and then later, my Daddy. I wanted to see them both again. I was certain they had come to visit because I was near death.

As I squinted toward the blinding light in the corner of the bedroom, trying to determine if I was hallucinating, I thought about the last days of my father's life in 1984. He had received a kidney transplant a year earlier but it failed rapidly. His body was rejecting the donated organ. I went to his hospital bedside in Lexington, Kentucky, but he was already going in and out of a coma. I wasn't certain if he recognized me, or knew I was there. My heart was aching. There was so much that had been left unsaid between us, for so many years. I wanted to bury my face in his shoulder and weep. I wanted Daddy to wrap his arms around me. I doubt he could have ever verbalized what was in his heart.

Daddy, like Mother, was a product of cold and distant parents. His father, Ogden Judd, never gave him any signs of affection and so my daddy had no experience of how he could show that he cared about any of us, although I know he did. He adored his granddaughters, Wy and Ashley, but his way of letting them know that he cared was to take out his wallet and hand them each a crisp twenty-dollar bill.

A couple of days before he passed away, I was sitting at the foot of his bed when his eyes slowly opened and he turned his head toward me. His final words to me were, "Honey, you look like a beautiful princess, sitting on a white horse." For that one moment in time I got to be a "Daddy's girl" again. I had wanted nothing more than to be his princess throughout my childhood. His opinion mattered more to me than anyone else's. He could uplift me with a nod of approval and devastate me with a frown. Most of what I tried to accomplish was in the hope that Daddy would feel proud I was his daughter. I tried so hard to carry the Judd banner with pride. I was hoping for a final connection that would heal the distance that had grown between us. As the Judds, Wy and I were starting to gain increasing popularity in the music industry. I wish that he had lived long enough to see our hometown of Ashland rename a public area the "Judd Plaza."

On the day of my father's funeral, Wy and I had to perform in Memphis. We were under contract and it was a sold-out venue. As soon as the funeral was over, we had to jump on our tour bus and hit the road to make our gig. I never had time to grieve for Daddy. That sorrow stayed unprocessed, shoved down into my subconscious, for years and years. But, like other memories, it was coming back to break my already grieving heart.

In desperation, Larry called Dr. Mona Lisa as a support system. He didn't know what else to do and he needed the insight from a professional who cared about me. After he and Ashley tried endlessly to get me to sit up and eat and to get out of bed and walk around, they admitted that they were out of options. As Larry described it to me later, he feared I was near death. My breathing was shallow and my skin was pale. I was very ill. Without jumping from the bridge, using a gun, or even pills, I was most certainly willing myself to die. Nothing seemed to matter to me. I had no regrets. I wanted to sleep away and never face my emotional pain again.

Larry called 911.

Chapter 9
The Cuckoo's Nest

I heard the ambulance siren screaming its way up our long driveway, but I was so disoriented I had no idea it was coming for me. Two medics followed Larry into our bedroom. They took my vital signs, tried to ask me questions, and radioed the results back to the emergency room doctor on call at our local hospital, Williamson Medical Center. I could hear them explaining that I was severely dehydrated and my blood pressure was only 80 over 50, but it still seemed like the foggy edge of a bad dream where you aren't quite awake, but not asleep, either. The medics were directed to give me an IV bag of a dextrose and saline solution.

Once the fluids circulated through my body, I was better able to comprehend what was happening. I had no intention of taking an ambulance ride. I didn't want the ER staff to see me in this pitiful condition, or have it be leaked to the tabloids. I had worked as a nurse at Williamson and I didn't want to have to face the humiliation of the staff I knew seeing me in this state of mind.

I didn't know what Larry had told paramedics on the way in, but when he left the room for a couple of minutes I told the paramedics a different story. I assured them that I had been suffering severe nausea and that I was dehydrated. I explained that I was a nurse and convinced them that I didn't need the emergency room;

I only needed a medication for nausea. I asked them to put Phenergan, a drug used for nausea and vomiting, into the IV. I convinced them that a bad flu had taken me out. After they checked in with the doctor, I got exactly what I wanted, a dose of Phenergan. I knew it would make me sleep. What the paramedics didn't know was that I wanted to sleep forever.

I may have been able to fool paramedics but, in the meantime, Larry and Ashley had consulted with Dr. Mona Lisa by phone and had come to the conclusion that I could no longer be the caretaker of my own mental health. They began to confer together about a plan for my rescue. I was too lethargic to even care, which was the most blatant clue that I needed someone else to take charge.

The next day, Dr. Mona Lisa arranged with Larry and Ashley for me to go into Vanderbilt Psychiatric Hospital for evaluation. She was still extremely worried that the Nashville psychiatrist had me on so many overlapping prescriptions that some of my issues were being caused by a chemical overload from the medications and my liver's ability to detox was maxed out.

There were often paparazzi near Vanderbilt University Medical Center just waiting to announce the next horrible downfall or emergency treatment of a celebrity. If they found out I was going to the psychiatric unit, it would be a free-for-all, especially because I was so mentally and physically exhausted that I'm sure I looked awful. For months I had never looked in a mirror if I could help it. It was a stranger staring back at me; someone I would have never become. But I was that stranger.

Ashley came up with a disguise for me to wear as a solution to avoid being caught by paparazzi in any unfortunate photos that I would always regret. The disguise was an ugly polyester plus-sized pantsuit, padded with pillow stuffing. I wore a curly dark brunette wig on my head, along with oversize dark sunglasses. The only thing I was missing was a trick-or-treat bag. I was unrecognizable.

For the first time in my adult life, I relinquished control. I had no idea what I was heading into, but I was absolutely terrified I was having a psychotic breakdown. Larry and Ashley carried me out to the car, where I lay down across the backseat so I wouldn't be seen. When we got to Vanderbilt, Larry drove up to a back door with no one around it, pulled the car up close to the door, and lifted me into a wheelchair.

Dr. Mona Lisa had called ahead, using her pull as a fellow psychiatrist, and arranged an emergency meeting with the chief of staff in charge of the psychiatric unit. I was so completely out of it, from being in bed for so many days, that I was babbling and gesturing, trying to communicate that I didn't want to be there. I was afraid and ashamed I was losing my mind.

The Vanderbilt psychiatrist saw how vulnerable I was and approached me with great kindness, treating me with respect and dignity. He got down on his knees, next to where I was seated, made eye contact, and promised he would listen to me no matter how tenuous my grip on reality was becoming. When he found out the number of different drugs I had been prescribed within the last year, he was appalled. He strongly suggested that I should go through a process of getting detoxed from the multiple antidepressants and benzodiazepines that were still in my system. I didn't really know what that would entail, but I surely knew, at this point, that I had no choice. My instincts told me I could trust this kind psychiatrist and I knew I had to stay in the psych ward, or else I was going to die.

I've done outrageous things in my life and have had many scary experiences, but I had never experienced the disbelief of being admitted to a psychiatric ward.

I was directed to a tiny eight-by-ten-foot room at the end of the hallway. I didn't expect what happened next, but I should have. The nurse assigned to my room took away everything that I came in with: my purse, my makeup bag, my costume, my regular clothing I was planning to go back home in, even the hairbrush and toothbrush I had brought. I was given a hospital gown to wear and a plastic cup for drinking water. I immediately begged Larry to take me back home. I told him that the dogs would be anxious about where I was. We had not been apart for more than a year, except for my time in Vancouver.

I hollered at Larry to find where they had taken my clothing and purse and bring it all back. He tried to calm my nerves by saying that it was the hospital protocol to take away all personal items, but that he would be there every day during visiting hours and would bring me anything I needed. I believed him. However, I still had no idea how I could remain in this hideous and impersonal room. The bed was only about eighteen inches off the floor. I knew the reason. It was a room set up for patients who were so out of it they might hurt themselves falling out of the bed. The window was coated with grime on the outside and it was hard to see anything through it. The walls had been painted the dreariest shade of mustard. There was no artwork, nothing that could be removed and used in a self-destructive way. Clearly, they didn't want patients to get too comfortable and want to stay.

*   *   *

I was terrified at the thought of Larry and Ashley leaving me there, but visiting hours policy had to be followed. After they had left, promising to be back the next morning, I sat on the low bed, slumped over, my head in my hands, sobbing.

When the Judds' career really skyrocketed and we would play to large sports arenas and auditoriums across the country, we would hire off-duty police officers at each venue as backstage security and to be on hand when we had our meet-and-greets, in case anyone became aggressive or pushy. We called these moonlighting officers our "cops du jour."

I've always had the highest respect for police officers, especially considering all the different experiences they must go through. I chatted with one female officer in Minneapolis and asked her out of curiosity, "What's your greatest fear?" She answered right away, "Being taken hostage." Then I asked her what title she held in her police department. She told me that she was a hostage negotiator. She then turned the tables, asking me about my greatest fear. I didn't even pause. "My greatest fear is not being able to take care of myself."

In the Vanderbilt psychiatric unit it appeared that my greatest fear was now a stark reality. I was feeling weak and at the mercy of the hospital staff. I was besieged by worry about being at the point of no return. What if the professionals here found me to be certifiably insane? Would they commit me for good? The doors on the insides of the psych ward were also locked. I couldn't leave even if I wanted to go. I felt claustrophobic and emotionally out of control. I thought, this is what jail must feel like.

I was assigned two nurses who would be in charge of me that night. As each one came in to check on me throughout the evening, I tried to make small talk, striving to sound as normal as possible. I wanted them to know that I was a nurse, too, so that they would view me as "one of them" and not a woman who had gone completely over the edge. One of the nurses reassured me in a serious and calm tone, promising, "You'll be okay. You're just someone who is overdue for some professional help."

I stared at the ceiling most of the night, listening to the sounds of the nurses conferring with each other in the hallway, the same way I used to do while working a shift as a professional nurse. I tried to remember the woman I used to be.

The next morning, the psychiatrist arrived early to meet with Larry and me to describe and get approval for the procedure used to get the overload of medications out of my system. He explained the serious method, calmly, as an everyday occurrence under his watch. I'm certain he never expected me to freak out the way I did.

The moment the doctor uttered the word phenobarbital, my anxiety spiked to the point where I began shaking uncontrollably. My teeth were chattering as I tried to cry out my objections. "I'm a nurse. I know what phenobarbital is!" Everyone tried to calm me down, but I remained terrified.

Phenobarbital is a highly dangerous drug that decreases brain activity and puts a person in a hypnotic state. Marilyn Monroe, Elvis Presley, and Margaux Hemingway all died from overdoses of phenobarbital. It's mostly used to bring relief to those with seizures and epilepsy. It depresses the nervous system, including breathing functions. Too much of it is deadly. In my case it would be used to help me withdraw from the multiple antidepressants and also the benzodiazepines I had long been prescribed. As it was explained to me, a fast withdrawal from certain medications like benzodiazepine can cause severe anxiety, agitation, an increased heart rate, and even seizures. Phenobarbital inhibits all activity in the brain, not just the unique set of receptors for anxiety or depression in a specific part of the brain. A specialist nurse sits at your bedside and takes your blood pressure every fifteen minutes, while very gradually the IV of pheno is started.

It must be carefully administered because it can cause your blood pressure to spike to the point of death. I had to sign many legal documents and have them witnessed, which indicates how dangerous this detoxing protocol can be.

I was assured that this was the most effective way to flush the multiple medications from my system and that I would be under constant surveillance. I knew this procedure would take my total compliance. I had to be in bed for the next thirty-eight hours while the strong barbiturate pulled the old drugs from my system. My apprehension was off the charts, but something had to be done to lower the toxicity of all the other myriad drugs in my body.

Soon after they started the procedure the nurses had to stop the IV flow of phenobarbital several times because my blood pressure would spike. I could see what was going on and it absolutely demolished any sense of feeling that I was in safe hands. I had no choice but to remain perfectly still, in my small, hard, and uncomfortable bed, continually scanning the faces of the nurses to see if they were calm or concerned.

Larry would come in to see me and sit on the other side of the bed to hold my hand. I wanted him to pull the IV from my arm and insist that he was taking me home, but I couldn't form the words to tell him. I felt as if I couldn't move under my own volition. I could tell that Larry was feeling nervous about this procedure, even though he would try to keep smiling at me. I felt the sensation of drops of water on the back of my hand. As I halfway opened my eyes to see where the drops were coming from, I realized Larry was crying.

In a state of forced immobility from the phenobarbital, my conscious mind took a forced siesta, allowing for long-buried thoughts from my subconscious to break through. I thought of one of my neighbors, a young married woman, from my early school-age years.

One morning, as we were getting ready for school, the phone rang. Mom was cooking breakfast, answered the call, turned off the burner under the scrambled eggs, and then flew out of the front door and straight across the street to the neighbor's house. My brothers and sister and I watched as a police car pulled up. Mother soon returned. She wouldn't tell us what had happened but was clearly very upset. Before I left for school, more cars pulled up in front of the neighbor's and then a Catholic priest hurried into the house.

As the weeks went by I would often see this young woman wandering around in her front yard, in the same wrinkled dress, talking to people who weren't there. My siblings and I would duck behind the hedge and watch her strange behavior, our hands over our mouths to suppress our inappropriate laughter. Then, one day she vanished. I finally asked my mother where our neighbor went. Mother very directly answered, "She had to go to a mental hospital. We will see if they ever let her out."

I nodded my head, as if I knew what she meant, but I was floored. I had no idea what a mental hospital could be, but it sounded like she probably didn't want to go. And, it seemed to be a place where they hid away hopeless people. It made me so sad and upset I went up to my room and just sat on the bed for a while, staring at the wall.

I found out that the young woman had lost her firstborn child to SIDS, sudden infant death syndrome. At that time, I had no reference point for understanding psychological issues, though I was surrounded with severe mental illness on both sides of my family. When you're a kid, you simply accept adults the way they are. Even though I could see that other families shared warmth and supported and encouraged one another, I didn't have any of that in my life. I didn't question what I was missing until I was an adult. I had never even heard the word *depression* until I moved to California at age nineteen. Once I understood what it meant, I wondered if Daddy might be a depressed person. I could never get him to laugh, even if I never saw him cry.

I never in a million years thought I would be depressed. Yet, here I was, involuntarily committed in a "mental hospital," wondering if my fate could be the same as my long-ago neighbor. Would they ever let me out? Was agreeing to this treatment the worst mistake of my life?

When the thirty-six hours passed, I was finally freed of the IV and having to lie still. However, following this treatment I was still having massive withdrawal symptoms from Klonopin, which has a half-life of up to sixty hours, meaning that the drug is still at half of its potency sixty hours after the last dose.

I was agitated and shaky and wanted nothing more than to go home to our farm and be outside in nature. To keep me in a calm state I was prescribed Seroquel, which snowed me under like a corpse in an avalanche. It's typically used as an antipsychotic drug but has also been given in a low dose to people with chronic insomnia to get them to a drowsy state. Oh, but it did so much more than keep me drowsy. It left me feeling paralyzed. I would have to crawl on my hands and knees into the bathroom. I had no sense of balance. Later I would read that one of the worst side effects is that it can paralyze the body and yet the brain remains alert.

I became completely immobilized by this powerful drug. Everything seemed to move in slow motion. I didn't bathe or brush my teeth. I lay on the bed for twenty-three hours a day, for over a week. I was very worried that I would get bedsores from being so inactive. I felt like my muscles were becoming weak and atrophied. I tried to take the nurse's hand and have her look at me as I mouthed the words "I'm in danger." She would only smile and pat my shoulder as if everything were normal. At one point, an RN looked down at me and gushed, "I love your music," which even then struck me as bizarrely inappropriate. I thought for a moment I might be hallucinating, but then I remembered how at Daddy's funeral a person asked me for an autograph. So, it happens.

I didn't know what time of day or night it was and I could only sense that Larry was by my side for every single visiting hour. I couldn't tell if it was the sun or the moon outside my dirty little window. He would bring me takeout food and help me sit up long enough to eat a few bites. I had truly lost hope that I would ever feel like a human being again. Dr. Mona Lisa flew to Nashville to check on my progress in person, and stayed on to be a support system for Larry and me.

After what seemed like years, yet was only nine days, I slowly began to be able to respond to the doctor. I was directed to go to group therapy at the end of the second week. It was a program called Activities of Daily Living. The first session, I attended in my nightgown. I still didn't have the energy or motivation to even run a brush through my hair. No one seemed to notice anyway. The other participants were all so depressed that they spent the hour staring at their feet. I'm certain that I looked like I needed this group class, but it wasn't a good environment for me. The therapist would monotonously take us through the steps of structured living: "Get up at the same time every morning, go outside, set appointments and keep them, force yourself into a schedule." It all seemed very kindergarten-simple and stifling to me. I hoped that I wouldn't ever be a person who could only stare at her feet.

The treatment staff of doctors and nurses could tell that I was on my way to functioning again when I was finally able to get up and take a shower and wash my hair. It felt like washing off layers of drug dependency that had latched on to my psyche like leeches, sucking from me all that used to be Naomi Judd. I didn't want the label of mentally ill or depressed person. I longed to have this nightmare behind me now, even though I didn't have a clue as to how I could really feel better. Well, I thought to myself, I will fake that I feel better; anything to get me out of this hospital situation. I begged Larry to take me home. But that wasn't about to happen. The psychiatrist informed me as he was signing my release forms that the real work had only begun. He recommended that I go directly into an intensive treatment program. He had contacted a rehab facility in Scottsdale, Arizona, where they would help me continue to detox from Klonopin. In addition, it was now time to deal with the trauma of my past, which had been making itself known through my panic attacks. This would take some time.

I didn't want to give it time. I was obsessed with getting to go home. Larry and Ashley felt differently. So did Dr. Mona Lisa. At a family conference with the Vanderbilt psychiatrist and his staff I heard that they all agreed that it was high time for me to take a long look at the legacy of mental illness in my family of origin and face all the dark secrets. They wanted me to be all the way well and not merely suppressing these shadows that had been displacing my sun for almost two years. I was still so buried under by Seroquel that I couldn't even speak to join their conversations regarding my future. With trepidation, I decided that I would have to comply with their wishes. After all, I thought, nothing could be more of a nightmare than this past month at Vanderbilt. I was dead wrong.

Chapter 10

The Trauma Egg

I ronically, the shell of the former Naomi Judd who left Vanderbilt Psychiatric Hospital was now entering an intensive month-long program in Scottsdale, Arizona, that implements a method of treatment starting with what's called the Trauma Egg, followed by other therapies.

Larry, Ashley, Dr. Mona Lisa, and the professional staff at Vanderbilt were well aware I would feel trapped and terrified by my lack of freedom if I had to live in another hospital environment. Any inpatient program was going to make me spiral downward, which is why they recommended the outpatient program in Scottsdale, Psychological Counseling Services. It was agreed that Larry and I would stay in a nearby inn together at night while I attended eight hours of daily therapy at their facility.

The therapists at PCS guided me to take a deep look at, and come to terms with, the curse of mental illness handed down from past generations. My personalized therapy plan was to begin by taking an inventory of past difficult emotional experiences and traumas that had shaped my personal belief system.

I learned that your current beliefs are based on your early life experiences and the memories and perceptions you have formed. On a large sheet of paper they had me draw an egg that represented a clean slate, me at birth. This is called the "Trauma Egg." Beginning with my very first memories of traumatic experiences, the therapist had me write them down chronologically from my earliest memory, at the bottom of the egg, continuing on to my current life.

My first traumatic memory that I put on the paper was of being sick with chicken pox and being molested by Uncle Charlie at Grandmommy Judd's house at age three and a half. As I ascended though my childhood years, other memories of molestation attempts by Uncle Charlie came to the surface of my consciousness. I had a difficult time writing them on the egg without my hands trembling. I had never told anyone in fifty-five years.

The next memory that returned to me was of being at my aunt Pauline's farm, Little Catt, at about age five. This was usually a place I felt safe, because it was in the middle of nowhere. There was no indoor plumbing, only a well in back of the house and a wood-burning stove in the front room used for heat. To bathe, we had to pump water from the well and then warm it on the woodstove. The outhouse was about fifty feet from the house and it sure was a long walk on chilly mornings. Aunt Pauline, a true Appalachian countrywoman, raised chickens, milked her cows, and had a big vegetable garden. She never went to a doctor. She grew herbs to use as medicine and made every meal from scratch. There was no such thing as a boxed cake mix at Aunt Pauline's.

As a child, my parents would allow me to stay with her for a week, especially during the summer. During those days I would rarely see another human being since Aunt Pauline's farm was on a rough dirt road. I would roam to my heart's content on the many acres of Catt Farm, singing to myself and making up fanciful stories, usually accompanied by one or two of Aunt Pauline's many dogs. I had invented an imaginary playmate named Elizabeth. She was angelic and lived in the dense woods at the edge of Aunt Pauline's property. She became a very real presence for me, assuring me that I was special and would make it in life. She said everything I wished my mother had said.

The interior of Aunt Pauline's house was as plain as an Amish homestead. No pictures adorned the walls, not even a single photograph of a family member. One simple calendar, given away free at the feed store every Christmas, hung on a nail. There were no rugs on the bare-wood plank floors. Every pot, pan, brush, and blanket in the house was something that was useful. I never saw a single knick-knack, flower vase, or decorative pillow in her house. Even the outside bird feeders were made from hubcaps that had dislodged from occasional passing cars when they hit the potholes on the dirt road in front of the farmhouse. Aunt Pauline would hammer the hubcaps to the top of the fence posts and fill them with suet for the cardinals. She would predict the weather by how much the cardinals were feeding and by what time the grazing animals headed for the barn.

If I heard a car on the road, I would run out of the house to see if it was someone who was going to stop. They would always just drive on by. Aunt Pauline preferred it that way. I didn't understand until I was well into adulthood that she was gripped by severe agoraphobia, as were three of her sisters: Evelyn, Ramona, and Faith. Only my father's fourth sister, Aunt Toddie, managed to escape the mentally ill Judd household, get married to a wonderful man, and raise her three kids, somehow bypassing the crippling emotional and mental problems of her sisters.

Aunt Pauline only went into town if absolutely necessary, which was about once a month for supplies. It was almost impossible for her to talk to people she didn't know very well. One day a truck did pull in at Aunt Pauline's farm. But it was no one I wanted to see. It was

Uncle Charlie. As he approached the house, I ran and hid, lying down between the rows of corn in the garden until he left. Later that week he came back again, but I wasn't aware of his arrival. I had no time to hide. I couldn't comprehend why Aunt Pauline wasn't afraid of him, too. She didn't seem to worry about having Uncle Charlie around. I couldn't possibly know that he wasn't interested in adult women, only tiny girls he could overpower, intimidate, and then threaten.

As soon as Aunt Pauline left the house to pull onions in the garden, Uncle Charlie came looking for me and cornered me in the bedroom. He tried to coax me toward him, like the friendly great-uncle. I remember being so confused, but I knew I couldn't trust him. I tried to bolt past him for the door, but he grabbed my arm. As soon as his hands were on me he tried to pull my clothes off.

Even though I was now only a kindergartener, I pointed at his face and squinted my eyes the way I had seen dueling cowboys do on the westerns Daddy loved to watch on TV.

"Don't touch me! I will tell my daddy. He has a gun. My daddy will kill you."

I have no idea how I had the moxie to make such a bold threat to him, but there was something inside me that knew cowering in fear wasn't going to help in the long run. I had to save myself, again. And I did. He let me go. I ran to the garden to be with Aunt Pauline. Once again, the adult who should have protected me didn't even notice I was trembling in fear.

Even my own mother and father never seemed to suspect I was emotionally terrorized every time I was in Uncle Charlie's presence. I recently found a photograph of me as a small child that brought back a fierce and chilling memory. I had been instructed by Grand-mommy Judd to stand next to Uncle Charlie for the photo. He has his arm on my shoulder, pulling me into his waist. My face is scrunched

up in disgust and my hands are clasped tightly in front of me, pro-
tectively across my lower half.

I later came to suspect that he had abused his own granddaughter. She was my age, but we went to different schools. I never met
her until we were teenagers. She approached me at a baseball game,
when our schools were playing against each other, and said, "Hi,
Naomi, I'm Susan, your cousin."

She was a beautiful girl with long, shiny black hair and high
cheekbones. As pretty as she was, she had the same haunted and
hunted look in her eyes that I often saw in my own. I felt, in my
heart, that Susan and I shared the same dark and sickening secret.
We never had any opportunity to talk, without other ears around,
but I would think of her often in the following years. Susan was shot
and killed in her home in the 1970s. Her case remains unsolved.

In the 1950s and '60s, the majority of parents never thought
about teaching their children how to protect themselves. No one discussed sexual abuse with kids. We now know the greatest danger
to young girls is from an adult they know, not a stranger. I often
thought that my mother might have suffered sexual abuse as a girl.
If she did, she would never say. Any experience that fell outside the
realm of the "all-American family" was "dirty laundry" that should
never see the light of day.

The common link among most of the traumatic events I wrote
down on the Trauma Egg during this therapy was my relationship
with my mother. Each painful memory shared a similar theme: being
exposed to a threatening or troubling situation and then having my
feelings go unrecognized or be dismissed by Mother.

The more I recalled from my early childhood, the more conscious I became of what formed my strongest and earliest lifelong
belief: that I couldn't trust her.

Another experience I wrote on the Trauma Egg was a full-fledged memory of coming close to being drowned at a city pool when I was six years old. The pool was a place for Mother to relax and have a lifeguard babysitter watch over my siblings and me.

I had been paddling around near the steps leading in and out of the water, minding my own business, when an older and much larger girl decided that it was my day to die. She grabbed my shoulders and plunged me under the water. When my head was near the bottom step, she turned around and sat down on it, grinding my face into the concrete stair. I was helpless. No one could see my arms and legs flailing about underwater. I knew the lifeguard wasn't watching the shallow end of the pool, where it wasn't over anyone's head. I felt the chlorinated water fill my nose, then pour into my throat. My vision began to go black and then I saw a bright white tunnel. My ears were throbbing with the pressure. I was drowning. I was going to die.

Once again, I used the only weapon I had, my fingernails. I dragged the tips of my fingers across the skin of her shins and then pinched her as hard as I could. Angry, the large girl stood up and I floated to the surface. I gasped for air as water poured from my nose and projected from my throat. I crawled up the steps and, on my hands and knees, lay down on the warm concrete until I could stand up. When I went to find Mother, sunning herself on her beach towel, I tried to explain to her what had happened. I wanted her to wrap me in the towel and comfort me. I wanted her to examine the scratches on my face and then be outraged enough to report the bigger girl. She only looked up at me long enough to scold, "Don't be dramatic."

Once again, she had failed to see I was in fear for my life. No sympathy or consolation would be coming from my mother. I wrapped myself in a towel and went to sit next to the lifeguard stand. I knew the bigger girl wouldn't risk picking on me within earshot of his authority. I sat there, a sad observer of other kids calling out to their mothers, "Mom, watch this!" as they did handstands underwater or cannonballs from the diving board. Their mothers watched. Their mothers smiled at them. I could only fantasize about what that would be like.

As my childhood progressed, one experience followed another that cemented the thought in my young mind that I was no more than an unimportant inconvenience to Mother. After taking a few years of piano lessons, which my daddy paid for, I played well enough to participate in the annual recital. I put on my favorite Sunday school dress and fixed my hair as best I could. I was certain that Mother would be pleased with my progress. I should have wondered if she would attend. She didn't, even though where I took lessons was only one block from our house. I was heartbroken.

On another occasion, the day of the grade school talent contest, I was brimming with enthusiastic energy about performing in the tap dance number I had learned in class. We waited for our music cue and then the curtain rose and the lights came up. My eyes scanned the faces in the audience, looking for Mother, as I tapped out the choreography the other kids and I had practiced many times. I guess I wandered too far near the edge of the stage in my attempt to locate my mother because when the curtain dropped at the end of the number, I was the only dancer left out in front of it. The audience broke into gentle laughter and I heard a few of the parents give me a sweet verbal encouragement as I turned up the charm, smiled, and waved, and "shuffled off to Buffalo" to the side of the stage where I could exit. After the show, some of the audience members gave me a hug and told me that it was their favorite moment of the talent show. I'm now convinced this was a turning point in my young life, that it set my destiny. I couldn't get Mother's personal attention, but I could get approval from an entire audience.

I couldn't believe Mother would miss something this important to me. My eight-year-old mind conjured a dramatic plot that she must have been kidnapped. I started to run home, imagining my mother being held hostage by some robbers, When I arrived home, Mother was where she could always be found, in the kitchen. I was crushed and confused. It wasn't that my mother had forgotten; it wasn't her priority. My mother didn't need saving, but my tender emotions did.

The junior high school I attended was more than a mile and a half from our house. During the winter months this became a problem. I didn't have a pair of boots, only one pair of low-heeled pumps that I had to wear every day. I would slip and slide through several inches of snow, which would seep over the edges of my pumps, freezing my feet. Some days would get so bad that I would stop at a friend's house along the way just to thaw my toes.

One morning there was a thunder and lightning storm that was blowing the rain almost sideways. Our old blue station wagon was always in front of the house, so I begged Mother to drive me to school. She refused. She never offered to drive me, even in the worst weather. I often arrived at school soaking wet or icy cold and would stand in the girl's bathroom trying to blot my wet hair with paper towels or warm my feet by the radiator.

As I continued to process each experience that was traumatic for me as a young girl, I uncovered an incredible amount of suppressed rage I had for the way Mother treated me. I wasn't aware that so much built-up anger lay under the surface of my psyche, but it now seemed to be erupting. One memory followed another. Each one contained the similar theme of being disregarded by my mother. My opinions, passions, personal taste, and emotions were all ignored with a shrug and her cliché answer of "That's just the way it is." I felt invisible and powerless.

One day I came home to find that Mother had decided to redecorate my bedroom. She had never mentioned her plan to me or asked my opinion about what I would like. For a girl who adored all things feminine and did my best to add flair to anything I owned, my new bedroom was like a slap in the face. Mother had picked out solid brown for everything: rug, bedspread, hideous plastic curtains, and a fake-wood laminated dresser. It looked like a cheap, generic truckers' motel room. Everything was practical without an ounce of style or personality. In contrast, my younger brothers' bedroom had a floral rug and bright-colored bedspreads that matched. It didn't make sense to me, but no one cared if I understood her reasoning. I had a good cry about it and then decided I just had to live with it.

Mother seemed to go out of her way to invalidate any effort I made at self-expression. When I was allowed to attend my first school dance, I spent hours getting ready. I was enjoying my popularity among my peers and I had looked forward to this social event for weeks. It was the sixties and a flipped-up bouffant, teased to a towering height, was all the rage. Of course, it wasn't a practical everyday style, but I wanted to make a good impression at my first dance. I layered and teased my hair to what I thought was perfection. I went into the kitchen to say goodbye to Mother as the boy I was going to the dance with arrived at the front door. Mother was canning pickles and turned from the counter to look at me. Silently, she picked up a mason jar full of sticky pickle juice and dumped it unceremoniously over my head. It was her way of disapproving of my grown-up style. I guess she thought words couldn't express her feelings. I sent Jimmy Keeton on his way and went upstairs to wash my hair. My first school dance would have to wait.

As an adult, looking back more than fifty years, each of these interactions with Mother felt like a purposeful attack on my growing sense of self. It was as if my mother was unconsciously, or perhaps very consciously, making certain that I knew that she was a depressed person and she was determined that I would be one, too. Recently, my youngest brother remarked to me: "I never understood why Mother treated you so differently than the rest of us."

It was the first time I had validation for my personal truth.

*   *   *

The competent therapists and staff at Psychological Counseling Services spent the first week helping me process the tumultuous emotions I had suppressed in my childhood. I was still having panic attacks almost every night. Vanderbilt may have detoxed my body from an overload of antidepressants and antipsychotics, but they left behind the depression and anxiety.

I finally learned about what was causing my panic attacks. My central nervous system had gone on overdrive from repressing bad memories for so many years. For me, the worst memories were of my childhood, feeling unheard and unloved.

One of the therapists explained that panic attacks are often based on lack of attachments. This was new information for me, but it didn't surprise me in the least. At one point, I was given two large poster boards to use to make a genogram, which is a family map. I was instructed to draw both sides of my family tree and write out significant personality traits of each family member and how I inter-

acted with them. A genogram is used to identify unhealthy relationship patterns in the family and helps reveal where dysfunctional
behavior and beliefs germinate.

As the clarity of who my relatives really were became visible
on the boards, I was also faced with my immediate anger over how
the abuse and trauma of decades of untreated mental illness was
destroying the next generation. As small children with little experience, each of us probably surmises that the way our family members behave is the way all adults are normally. In my circumstance,
I didn't have one single family role model who reflected a mentally
healthy attitude through the stages of life.

The therapist worked with a professional who specialized in
genealogical signs of mental illness. When he looked over my genogram, he couldn't believe it. He called in another expert to help him
study my history. My grandparents, aunts, and uncles on both sides
were all deeply peculiar and ran the gamut of emotional disorders
from agoraphobia to obsessive-compulsive, from extreme narcissism
to pathological issues that rendered them unable to function in any
regular social circumstance.

On my mother's side, my great-grandmother and all of her adult
children lived in a closed-up, dark, cigarette-smoke-filled house.
They were rarely seen in public, outside of working at the Hamburger Inn, the restaurant managed by Grandma Burton. No one
ever smiled or laughed in that house. Daddy's sisters, except for my
aunt Toddie, all had their dysfunctional quirks, superstitions, and
paranoia that kept them isolated from society. They were reclusive
and compelled to follow their established routines, never extending
themselves beyond their comfort zones. I tried to charm them into
smiling and coax them into the daylight or out for an adventure,

anything I could think of to bring them joy, but they never responded. Not one of them ever gave me a gift, played a game with me, or even took me to the city park across the street from where I grew up.

When I was out on tour, I would send my aunts letters and post-cards from various cities. I would stop by to see them in Kentucky if I was anywhere in the region. Daddy always appreciated that they seemed to lighten up a bit when I was around. I put a lot of energy into making them feel I cared about them. But it was rarely returned. They would stiffly hug me hello and goodbye, but that was it. No one ever told me they missed seeing me or made any inquiry about how I was doing. Filling out the information for these family boards with some of the counselors helped reveal to me what my aunts truly were: profoundly depressed and self-absorbed agoraphobics, with obsessive-compulsive disorders.

Aunt Pauline never married. She never went to see a doctor or dentist. Her hair went completely gray in high school. Once Grand-daddy Judd bought her the farm property, she moved there and never left or traveled anywhere else her whole life.

Aunt Evelyn could not function socially at all. She never went on a date and had no friends. She stayed inside, by herself, compulsively cleaning the house all day long.

Aunt Ramona had a possible chance at a normal life when she found employment on an army base. There she met a man and got married. But she never extended her life beyond that. She had to stick to a specific routine and not waver, such as only going to the grocery store at 5 p.m. on Fridays. None of them would even go to church.

When each one of them, Pauline, Evelyn, Ramona, and Faith, died, she had no one to attend her funeral. Not one of them had a sin-gle friend. The love I felt for them was futile because they couldn't access their own emotions. I was surprised when a long-repressed truth rose to the surface. I had hateful feelings for my aunts when they were all dead. My memories of being subject to their mental illnesses made me furious at my own parents. But what could I expect? My parents were cut from the same cloth and made little effort to change the way they were treated as children in how they treated their own kids. Daddy was never spontaneously affectionate to any of us, although I longed for his attention even more than Mother's. As a child, I knew the exact sound of his pickup truck coming down the street and would run to the front gate to meet him. I'd attempt to throw my arms around him, but that would usually result in a fast hug as he brushed by and headed inside for his dinner. Every Friday night I would watch boxing on TV with Daddy, even though the sight of the fighters' swollen faces made me wince.

I would take any opportunity to spend time with him. I was a "daddy's girl," which, looking back, didn't mean that much, except in my own mind. He never gave me any special attention or privileges. The only time I had physical contact with him was when I got a whipping, which would happen with the slightest misbehavior, anything he considered a public humiliation.

I always had honor roll grades on every report card. It was expected, but luckily I've always been an enthusiastic learner. One year, in junior high, a teacher wrote "whispers in class" on everyone's report card in the comment section, even though I had an A in her class, too. Daddy was furious that I received any unfavorable comment and got his belt ready.

At a very young age I found a pain-free way to receive my punishments. My mother had a very thick rubber girdle with plastic stays sewn into it. It was so sturdy it could stand up on its own. I would tell Daddy that I had to use the bathroom. Then I'd sneak into Mother's dresser drawer and pull the girdle armor on under whatever I was wearing. I never felt one lash of the belt, but I certainly hollered and carried on as if I did. Since Mother always thought I was "being dramatic" about everything, I figured I might as well live up to her description. Following the whipping, I'd return the girdle to the drawer and go on my merry way.

The last whipping I got was at age seventeen. I had gone on a double date to a movie at the local theater. We missed the start time of the first movie and waited for the second show, which caused me to be late for my curfew. I was only hoping the boy who dropped me at my front door couldn't hear Daddy telling me to get ready for a whipping. It's the last time the girdle came to the rescue. But the damage to my self-esteem was far more painful than any stripe his leather belt would have made.

In hindsight, I only had two ways of knowing that my father loved me or was proud of me: He paid for me to have piano lessons and he taped my school picture to the cash register at his gas station for all of his customers to see. Every time I went to his gas station, I would check to make sure my picture was still there. I think I didn't take my father's lack of affection personally because I never saw him display any affection to my mother, either. Daddy only once took Mother out to a movie, *The Bad Seed.* They never invited other adults over, even though Mother's cooking would have left them wanting to return.

I'm not sure that any of the three generations of mothers on my mom's side ever produced a drop of oxytocin, which is the chemical messenger produced in the brain when a mother is bonding with a newborn baby. Not surprisingly, my lack of attachment to my mother stems from her lack of love and connection to her own mother, Edie Mae.

In Scottsdale I learned that the first attachment to a child's primary caregiver is the most important relationship in life. By the time the child is age three, the brain is already 85 percent developed. This early relationship with the mother and father sets up a person's emotional patterns and even biological foundation. Holding, kissing, smiling, and laughing all create specific neurochemical activity in the child's brain. This leads to healthy brain systems and gives a child a solid foundation for future relationships and attachment. Lack of attachment or bonding with a parent can have long-term repercussions for the child. It can take years to repair the emotional damage from early neglect. Sometimes the damage can't be undone. Many who lack that early bonding grow up to be adults who rarely feel secure in their relationships and can suffer depression and panic disorders. It became clear to me that my own strong attachment to my daughters came from my determination that they feel loved and treasured for who they are.

There were times I failed as a mother when they were young, but I have to accept that I had had no support system on a day-to-day basis, no partner who was active in their lives, and had not learned good parenting skills from my own mother and father. However, my motivation was always to give them a good future with many opportunities.

Each session with the therapists uncovered new damaging evidence that I had never had a family who loved, encouraged, or protected me. I had toughened up at a very young age and found my own way, but even success won't fill the deep hole left in the psyche when a child grows up in an unsafe atmosphere, rarely being affirmed or even acknowledged by the adults in her life.

When Larry would return to the center to pick me up at dinnertime, I would be emotionally drained. He was gentle and didn't ask many questions. He would figure out some type of food for us to carry out and take back to the inn. I still didn't want to be seen in public. I didn't want anyone finding out about my severe depression and anxiety. "Look, Harold. There's that crazy Naomi Judd. What a shame!"

On a couple of evenings, Larry and I went for a long drive in the car and sang along with the radio. I would look out the window at a landscape that was endlessly the same: parched brown desert, dotted with sharp-edged succulent plants or cacti that could pierce one's skin. It seemed like a reflection of my internal landscape, barren and colorless, with painful, knife-sharp memories. Would the search for my mental well-being ever end?

Chapter 11

Reliving the Past

I was emotionally exhausted and wanted to go home at the end of my first week of intensive outpatient therapy. I had cried many times in the previous seven days and I thought I had no more tears to shed and had come to grips with the memories. The therapists discovered that I was suffering from post-traumatic stress disorder and had been for most of my life. The accumulation of repressed negative emotions over the years was now taking its toll on my sanity and sense of well-being. As one therapist advised me, "Your subconscious is trying to get your attention now. It's screaming that you have to pull these memories up. Look at them in the light of day. You must finally realize how they are negatively affecting your present. Talk about it all."

Larry also thought it was a good idea for me to continue on and process more of my post-traumatic stress disorder. I thought, Therapy is nothing like a concert tour. You can't move on to the next city and a whole new atmosphere the next day. Therapy is more like an archaeological dig. You have to persistently move the surface aside to get at what's underneath. Most of what you find may be broken, with sharp edges, so often it feels painful or hopeless. But you have to stay with it to excavate and analyze the specifics of what really happened in your past and how that has influenced your mental health today. I agreed to stay on track.

The next morning, as I was getting dressed I thought about my next-door neighbors when I was growing up, Cecil and Mary Agnes. They were a salt-of-the-earth-couple. Cecil ran the chicken hatchery in Ashland. They had three daughters who were my play-mates and they always included me. When I was at their house Mary Agnes would say, "I have four daughters." She and Cecil were both very affectionate and would hug me as much as they did their own girls. I cherished their attention. I found every opportunity I could to spend time at their house, which I knew as well as my own. Long after I left Ashland, Mary Agnes would send me cards saying how proud she was of my success. Whenever I would give an acceptance speech at a country music award show or the Gram-mys, I would always picture Cecil and Mary Agnes, sitting on their blue floral couch, watching me. The last time I saw the two of them was when I was the grand marshal in the Ashland Fourth of July parade. I was sitting up on the backseat of an open con-vertible, waving to people lining the sidewalks. Something caught my eye in the doorway of our church and I turned to look. It was Cecil and Mary Agnes, smiling and waving at their fourth daugh-ter. Even across the heads of a dense crowd, their genuine affec-tion reached out to me and captured my heart. I contemplated how my life would have turned out if I had been their actual daughter. Would I have memories that made me pace the floor almost every night after waking up with a panic attack?

*   *   *

Through an additional therapy called EMDR (eye movement desen-sitization and reprocessing), I delved into the traumas that came from feeling a lack of attachment. EMDR is a therapy technique that uses the natural way our eyes move in REM sleep to process traumatic feelings and memories that our brain is unable to process during sleep, which is when we are usually able to resolve our feelings about an experience. However, if the experiences are extreme and traumatic they get stored in the nervous system and repressed from our consciousness. They are still there, inside of us, along with every sight, sound, and smell associated with the traumatic experience, and can replicate the original stress response every time they surface. These unprocessed emotions and memories create disturbances in the normal function of emotions. EMDR is seen as breakthrough therapy in unlocking the traumatic memory and moving it out of the nervous system and into a normal memory that isn't fraught with the original feelings of danger.

As it turns out, I have many, many memories that I had locked away because, for much of my life, I had no way to express my emotions to someone I could trust. Most of my memories were heavy and traumatic, but they don't have to be. Even something that appears to be a simple life experience can hold a feeling of trauma that gets suppressed. For example, it could be an incident as fleeting as being embarrassed in front of the classroom once as a child. No one else remembers it, but you may have stored it away and it still affects your belief system about your intelligence.

I was able to process some traumas that I had remembered for many years, but whose ability to affect me I thought I had gone beyond.

The worst memory to process through EMDR was finally dealing with a horrible time when I was so desperate to have the feeling of being loved by someone, I unwittingly put my children and myself in a path of danger I honestly didn't see coming. My shame about this time period, in my mid-twenties, was so overwhelming I had pushed it far down into my subconscious. Even though I had spoken of it in public once or twice, in sympathy with women who needed sheltering from abuse, it was as if I were telling someone else's story, certainly not my own. I had never processed the lasting trauma of being punched, hit, and raped by a guy on heroin whom I dated in 1972.

Unbeknownst to me, he had bipolar disorder, which I had no clue about until years later, when I had more understanding of various mental illnesses. Early on in the relationship, he was full of love and passion, a talented artist and poet, and very protective and attentive to Wynonna and Ashley. In my fantasy, he was a charming knight in shining armor. Then, after a period of time, the gate started to swing in a different direction and he became full of jealous rage for a day or two. At first I thought it was a temporary insecurity since the relationship was new, but then the gate was blown right off the hinges. He began to stalk my every move at work and home, getting verbally aggressive and physically abusive by hitting me several times when he was convinced I was seeing another man, which I wasn't.

Even though I had begun to be terrified of him, I abruptly ended the relationship. He trailed me constantly, leaving me threatening notes where he was certain I would find them. For a short period of time, I didn't hear from or see him, so I thought my nightmare might be over. Then there was the heart-stopping moment I pulled into my driveway and saw in the rearview mirror that he was carrying boxes into the apartment directly across the street. He had rented the place so he could watch my house day and night from his balcony. I was petrified that he would kidnap one of my girls to get my attention. They couldn't understand why I rarely allowed them to play outside.

One night the phone rang at 2 a.m., waking me up. He was on the line, saying that he had Wy in his possession. I couldn't breathe. She had begun sleepwalking occasionally and had managed to open the front door, sound asleep, and head down the sidewalk toward Sunset Boulevard. Because he was stalking my apartment, he saw her come out onto the porch.

I was grateful he didn't hold her hostage and returned her safely to my arms. I thanked him, with my knees shaking in fear, still finding it hard to reconcile my feelings from when I thought he was a safe person in my life with the monster he had become. As a master of manipulation, he tried to use the incident as a bargaining chip, asking to come inside the house. It didn't work on me anymore. There was no turning back. I recognized fully what an unstable person I had allowed into my life. I never wanted to see his face again. I shut the door quickly and double-locked it. I didn't sleep the rest of the night as he sat on the porch talking to me through the locked door.

I could never feel safe, again, and one sleepless night followed another. I knew I would have to relocate as secretly as I could, but I didn't have the money for a security deposit on a new apartment.

I started to pick up some modeling jobs, after my day job, to put away a little cash to be able to move away. Then, one evening, when the girls were spending the night with our neighbor and my new friend, Nancy, and her little girl, Gabrielle, because I had a modeling gig that ran late, I arrived home to find that he had broken into my house and was hiding out and waiting for me to return.

When I walked into the house, he grabbed me and smashed my face into the wall. Then he dragged me around the house by my hair, while he rummaged through everything I owned, spilling the contents of my purse out onto the floor, overturning drawers, and pulling everything out of the closet, looking for proof I was seeing other men. After that he threw me down hard onto the wood floor, and using his booted foot stomped on my torso, then ripped my clothing and raped me.

I only escaped when he went into the kitchen to shoot up another vial of heroin. He overdid the dosage and passed out. I ran to Nancy's apartment and pounded on the door. She saw my bruised and battered face and torn clothing and wouldn't let me stay. She was afraid he had followed me there and would pick up where he left off, beating her, too. I knew she felt badly about it, but truthfully, she had warned me about him from the start. I should have listened.

I gathered up my two sleepy little girls and drove to a nearby motel in West Hollywood. I had no money or identification with me. The kind night clerk could see that I was in bad shape and afraid for my life and gave me a key to one of the smaller rooms, where the girls and I huddled together in one full-sized bed. They had no idea what I had been through or why I couldn't stop trembling. After the girls were asleep, I walked the two blocks to the West Hollywood sheriff's station. A kind sheriff named Al, who had become a friend to my girls and me after I met him earlier in the year, was there. I reported the rape and assault. He looked up my attacker in his files, made a few phone calls, and found out he had a long police record and convictions in Oklahoma. Al offered to take me to a hospital, but I had to go back to be with my daughters. Other policemen went to my home, but found it empty.

The next day, I had no choice but to go to my job as a receptionist. I couldn't afford to lose a day of pay. I was barely getting by. I dropped the girls off at their schools and drove by the house to see if it was still safe to go in for clean clothes. His car wasn't anywhere to be seen, so I dashed inside to wash my face and put foundation powder over the bruise near my left eye. I didn't have time to pick up the mess left behind, including my destroyed sense of safety, which I would carry with me after the rape no matter where I went. I had to put my actions on automatic pilot. I had to go to work. I had to make enough money for my daughters to have food, clothing, and health care. My own physical and mental well-being was not even on the list of priorities.

I couldn't take the time to get myself much-needed help; that had become the story of my life. There were no mental health services or shelters for battered women that I knew of. I was alone and voiceless, once again.

I couldn't tell anyone about this brutal rape, so I pushed the horrible event out of my mind as I devised the plan to get my girls and myself out of Los Angeles. Al was concerned and warned me that my attacker, who I sensed was stalking me daily, might try to kill me if I didn't leave town. I knew he was right.

As soon as I could, and though I had very little money and no family support, I escaped with my daughters to live in a remote hunting and fishing cabin at the end of Daniel Boone road outside of Lexington, Kentucky, and enrolled in my first year of nursing school. The harassment didn't stop, as he continued to send threatening letters to my mother's house for years after, trying to locate me.

But now, forty-five years later, while going through EMDR therapy, it all came back to life in vivid and horrifying high definition.

Every unresolved and unexpressed emotion of that trauma remained buried in my nervous system. I thought I had covered it well with denial, but it was all still there. More than the physical damage and pain of the rape, I had been carrying the shame and self-blame of this crisis for my entire adult life. Because I had no one to turn to when it happened, it became a dark secret and a source of gut-wrenching amount of guilt that I had exposed my children to a criminal. It was the 1970s and if a woman was sexually assaulted there was a high chance of her being judged, stigmatized, and blamed. In addition, police apathy toward women who reported rape was at an all-time high. Even today, 6 percent of women who don't report being raped say it was from fear of having the police not believe them.

During my time at PCS, with the help of the therapists, I gained an understanding of how past emotional and physical traumas can go relatively unnoticed for years, especially when you are completely involved with your work, your kids, and staying safe and healthy. When I was in my twenties and thirties, I would drop from exhaustion into bed and sleep, without even dreaming, through the four or five hours I had before the alarm went off. I was exhausted in mind and body from working long hours, attending nursing school, trying to keep up whatever meager living arrangements we had, taking care of the girls, and squeezing in one or two hours to study. There was no time for self-reflection. I had no idea there was such a thing as therapy.

When things slow down a bit and you have time to yourself, the disturbing symptoms of past traumas arise from the subconscious. As uncomfortable as it is, there is great healing value in looking at every possible source of traumatic experience in your past. I can testify that it's not subtle or easy. I had learned to run the obstacle course of my psyche over the years, never slowing down to remove the obstacles instead of jumping over or going around them.

The most healing benefit of doing intensive therapy in the program at PCS was having my personal feelings finally validated by their therapists and staff. It's so important to be able to verbalize feelings and memories to someone who is neutral and trained in dealing with trauma. I felt I was in a safe environment where I could speak freely without censoring myself to protect the feelings of family or friends. It was a relief to talk to a therapist who could guide me, and who truly understood how seriously frightening it is to be encased in depression and anxiety that you can't control.

I was a creative and expressive child born into a family that couldn't acknowledge and accept any show of vulnerability. I was shut down every time I had even the smallest expression of longing for family warmth. As a child, I always longed to celebrate special occasions or family traditions, anything to make our very routine home life more interesting or special. Mother owned one decorative tablecloth that we would use only on holidays. The tablecloth made our everyday dinnerware seem a bit more special.

One Thanksgiving, when I was about twelve years old, I offered up this suggestion as we gathered for dinner: "Why don't we go around the table and say what we are each grateful for." My idea met with blank stares from both my parents and my siblings. Then Daddy blandly wondered out loud, "Why would we do that?" He put a forkful of mashed potatoes in his mouth and everyone else followed his lead, eating in silence. I understood that matters of the heart were not to be discussed. It was a message I never forgot.

When I was first at PCS and the therapists were describing the Trauma Egg and how to recall specific childhood traumas, the initial thought that went through my head was, Why in the world would I do that? It was a question permanently burned into the part of me that feels I have very few people to trust. If, at age twelve, I couldn't share what I was grateful for with the people who supposedly loved me, how could I possibly share my hurts and sorrows with strangers? I would have to learn to trust again. It would be a bridge I needed to cross for my own self-awareness and peace of mind. The alternative was finding a bridge to jump from.

None of it was easy. At the end of each week I would want to go home to Tennessee. I was tired of delving into my past, even though I had only processed the first few decades of my life. The therapists at PCS pleaded with me to stay, reminding me: "How do you think you got here? Panic disorder is destroying your life and you're really not out of the woods yet."

At the end of the fourth week, I convinced myself that I was stable enough to get back to real life. I will process the rest of the trauma and emotions on my own, I promised the caring staff. I guess that's like saying to a surgeon, when you're the patient under anesthesia, "Thanks, I'll stitch myself closed." It doesn't work that way. All wounds must heal from the inside out. Wounds that haven't been completely cleaned out are prone to infection, more pain guaranteed.

Chapter 12

The Last Dirty Secret

Tere is no psychiatrist in the world like a puppy licking your face," author Ben Williams once said, a line often quoted by dog lovers around the world. If only the joy my dogs expressed at my homecoming and the happiness I had at reuniting with them after two months away could have continued endlessly, I would have been healed forever. I had missed them so much.

Dogs display an unconditional love that has no boundaries. Our pets can sense the energy depletion when you're struggling with physical or emotional issues and they try with their natural empathy to help us heal ourselves. That's why therapy dogs are so popular in hospitals, rehabs, and even hospice as a source of deep comfort. My rescue dog, Maudie, will lie on top of me if I'm upset or scared.

I'd longed for the privacy and peace of my own home. I didn't want to attend any more group therapy sessions or dredge up more experiences of my past. I ached to return to my cozy kitchen couch and be mentally consumed in true crime TV shows or more reruns of *Law & Order*. I successfully ignored my intuition, which whispered persistently, "You can't escape the repressed emotion buried deep within your core. It will erupt sooner or later."

But I was going to try like hell to escape it all. I steeled myself to win against this debilitating foe, determined to drive my depression and anxiety out of my mind.

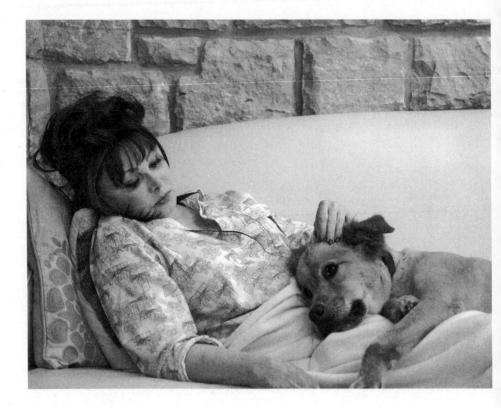

The peace at Peaceful Valley was temporary. One morning, not long after I came home, we received a phone call from our financial auditors and our law firm. My lawyer regretted to inform me that it was obvious that a previous business associate we had worked with had managed to pilfer $3 million from our income in royalties and fees over the course of a number of years. I had always made the decisions on how to handle the Judds' career income. Wynonna never asked about finances and if I tried to include her in the process she would say that all she wanted to do was sing. She was young, but that's the time when it's good to get into the habit of knowing what's going on in your money world.

It's an age-old story about performers and slick business partners who take them to the cleaners; I never thought it would happen to me. Usually, when this kind of story breaks in public, people shake their heads and wonder, How did they let that happen?

When you're a performing artist, you have to trust other people to help you manage all the elements of your career because your income is from many different sources. Unfortunately, I trusted the wrong guy. Going from abject poverty in the 1970s to making lots and lots of money in the 1980s was an unbelievable dream come true. I appreciated every fan who bought a concert ticket and every record sold. I took nothing for granted.

I almost collapsed on the floor after hearing that I had been scammed so badly. Larry had to manage the rest of the call, during which the lawyer wanted to know if I would press charges. He said I could have this immoral cheat imprisoned for eight to ten years. We told him we would get back to him soon.

Once it was known among those who work with me, people came out of the woodwork to tell me of their suspicions all along. Even Larry admitted that he had a "bad feeling" about him. As I understand it, I didn't pick up on the clues because he put on such a good show of professionalism when I was around.

Larry and I had an intense talk about how to proceed with this disastrous new information. I was devastated and probably should have been furious, but in my depression I could barely stand to think about the effort it would take to prosecute him. I couldn't face what it would mean to have to dig up so many facts and round up witnesses. The lawyers said that the court system could take years. I had never used a lawyer for anything other than to look over my entertainment deals. I had never been to court, even for a traffic ticket, because I've never had one.

Larry understood my position completely. We decided to let it go. However, I did have the message delivered to the perpetrator, loud and clear, that I knew of his thievery and could put him away for ten years. I wanted him to be constantly looking over his shoulder.

After being punched in the gut by this news, my panic attacks came raging back in full. I couldn't lie flat in bed because it felt like a suffocating coffin. At first I propped my head and shoulders up with many pillows, but then Larry decided to order one of those reclining beds that can be adjusted to elevate your head or feet, but it only brought a little relief. When my exhausted brain finally relaxed enough to doze off I would suddenly gasp as if I couldn't catch my breath. The fright of feeling as though I couldn't take a deep, natural breath would bring on a panic attack in full. I began to spend three or four hours pacing the hallways once more. I cleaned out and organized every drawer in the house. I took everything out of the kitchen cabinets and cleaned the shelves.

I also found myself a prisoner to a new bothersome phobia: fear of the dark, nyctophobia. I had to have the bathroom light left on all night so I could see everything in the bedroom. I didn't want to be left alone at night, ever.

Each panic attack would crash over me, bringing increasing shortness of breath, tingling and numb arms and sometimes legs, flushed skin, cold sweat, a feeling of being physically choked, and surge after surge of adrenaline through my veins. The despair of feeling that this level of anxiety could be with me for the rest of my life was profound, even beyond tears. Anxiety at that level impairs your judgment of what is reality and what is not. I couldn't think clearly, sometimes for hours and hours on end.

It was during a particularly harsh night of internal terror when I remembered that I had stashed Klonopin in secret places around the house before I was hospitalized in the psych unit at Vanderbilt. It suddenly seemed like a lifeline as I was being pulled under by my panic disorder. I found a packet, hidden out of Larry's sight, and took one. My body and mind became more relaxed, as if I had spent the day in physical exertion and could now sit down on a sandy beach and watch the waves come in. My blood pressure became consistent and my throat relaxed enough for me to be able to breathe deeply. I didn't even care what extremes I had been through to get the drugs out of my system. I only wanted relief. Klonopin gave me a feeling of mindless calm, and I questioned why I ever needed to be off of it.

As fall rapidly approached, bringing shorter days and gray skies, I had a harder time rallying the enthusiasm I had had about recovering on my own when I left Scottsdale. Larry made sure my "Happy Lights" were turned on in the kitchen before I had a cup of coffee every morning. I had already owned one Happy Light for a few years, since I had already been diagnosed with seasonal affective disorder, or "wintertime blues."

Happy Lights are full-spectrum light boards that replicate the effects of daylight and are supposed to recalibrate the body's natural cycles. People who use the lamps have reported an increase in energy and focus and an improved mood. Larry ordered two more lamps to add to the kitchen counter, hoping that the light would improve my emotional state. I don't know how I would have managed without them as the fall turned into a foggy swamp of thick, gray days where the sun retreated for weeks on end. I have recommended them to all of my friends who live in overcast parts of the country.

Ashley would come by to see me almost every afternoon that she was in town. She would find me, in my usual spot, under a blanket, with my dogs, on the kitchen couch. I could see that my long-running depression and anxiety were having an effect on my daughter. She had never experienced a panic attack and tried hard to understand what I was going through. I knew Ashley would never be someone who would tell me to "get over it," because she has walked her own path through a long-standing depression she has been able to rise above. She gives me hope for my own ability to overcome the family illness.

In 2006 she underwent almost six weeks of treatment for depression. As Ashley told Matt Lauer on the *Today* show, "I'm very happy to talk about it because, for me, when I talk about it, it helps me to reduce my own shame. I've been so blessed with finding a solution that how dare I not share that solution with others that face challenges? There's still a lot of stigma and taboo around something that's perceived as a mental illness."

I was now feeling the "shame" my daughter had revealed years before and had talked about on TV shows and in print media. I wanted to be able to function as myself again, but I had lost trust in my own reactions and was concerned about being in public, where I might embarrass myself. My reputation of being a person who gives comfort and hope to anyone struggling with an illness was at stake. When a person has a visible physical disability, such as a missing limb, cerebral palsy, or blindness, people react in ways that accommodate the person, making certain she is taken care of and not left to fend for herself. No one can "see" your depression or anxiety, so people expect you to function normally, when the reality is that normal functioning is not possible.

Ashley knew that going to a restaurant or being in a social situation would be hard on me, but she was still on a daily mission to get me off the kitchen couch. She would bundle me into my long coat and make me go outside for fresh air. After we had walked around the meadow a couple of times we would sit under the giant oak tree while she held my hand. Ashley has always found a sense of God in nature and appreciates any opportunity to combine physical exercise with a beautiful natural setting. She would regale me with tales of her experiences hiking in the Smoky Mountains or an intensive yoga retreat in the piney coastal mountains of Big Sur, California, anything to connect me to real-life moments.

I would listen intently, but I couldn't imagine how I would be able to enjoy life that much ever again.

I'm grateful Ashley is such a free spirit and open to new experiences. From the time she could understand my words, I've told her she's special and can do anything. She believed me, and I like to think that has helped shape her life. Ashley recently got her master's degree in global economics from Harvard and is now at the University of California, Berkeley, studying for her PhD.

I wasn't sure if Wynonna was aware that I hadn't been home for two months. Ashley never let her know. Through therapy, Ashley has developed and maintains excellent boundaries. She chooses to not get involved in my relationship with Wy, and I respect her for that. I didn't tell Wy about being hospitalized because I felt in my bones that if she knew the extent of my depression and panic disorder and the treatments I was undergoing it would affect her, too. She's as impressionable and emotional as I am. I didn't want her to start feeling a symbiotic panic or depression.

As November approached, the police chief from the city of Manchester, Tennessee, asked me to host the upcoming Veterans Day presentation on the courthouse steps. I would present military swords of recognition to about ten local veterans. Though I was feeling worse than ever, I knew I would never forgive myself for turning down this request. I think Veterans Day is one of the most underappreciated holidays in our country and that it should be held in the highest esteem. It would be a good idea to require all school-aged children to attend a ceremony like this one so that they are aware of the loyalty and sacrifice made by brave citizens who put their lives on the line for our freedoms. I was deeply honored to be able to have a chance to shake their hands and thank them in person.

The day arrived, and the sun broke through the clouds as a crowd gathered near the steps of the courthouse. A bagpipe player added to the solemn atmosphere with his stirring, mournful music.

When it came time for me to present the commemorative swords, I read aloud each name inscribed on them. All were men, except for one woman. I couldn't believe the name of that woman: Althea Cimino, a beautiful nurse who had served in the Korean War.

Althea had been my nursing supervisor when I worked multiple shifts in the ICU at a local hospital in the early 1980s. She was my mother's age and I adored her for encouraging me with her bright smile every day at work. She and I had a cherished relationship. She allowed for my high-spirited approach dealing with patients and appreciated how I threw myself into my job. She also got my sense of humor and would only feign disapproval when I caused other nurses to shriek in cascades of laughter at the nurses' station. Our jobs were stressful eight hours a day, so a two-minute laugh break was our release, and Althea understood that. I was grateful to her for helping me arrange my schedule to be able to get in enough hours to support my children and also have time to shop Wynonna's and my audition tape where and when I could. Once the record deal with RCA was signed, I knew that it was time to focus full-time on music, and when our first song was getting airtime on the radio, I decided to move on from nursing.

When our first hit song, "Mama He's Crazy," went to number one, I received a letter in the mail from Althea. She wrote about how proud she was of me along with compliments about my "real pretty" singing voice. It meant the world to me. Since 1984, we had exchanged Christmas cards through the mail every year, with her recounting the times she saw me on TV and filling me in on her five children. I had not laid eyes on her since my last day on the nursing job.

I burst into tears when I presented her sword to her. She still had the exact same smile and spirited personality. Her five grown children had flown in to be there as the city of Manchester honored her.

After the ceremony, Althea invited me to her home for a celebration lunch with her children. She had already prepared her famous chicken salad.

She was now a widow, but still lived in the house her husband built. Every wall held framed photos of family occasions over the years. In her basement was a playroom for the grandchildren along with a closet full of dress-up costumes. No one would ever question that this was the home of a happy and emotionally stable family.

As we toured her house, Althea held my hand or put her arm around my waist. Her adult children all hugged me and made sure I was comfortable. In the time span of that two-hour lunch, I felt more maternal and familial affection and warmth from Althea and her children than I had in my entire childhood from my own mother and siblings. Even though it had been a beautiful reunion and afternoon, I felt my heart sink with the hopeless longing to have this type of relationship with my own mother.

The following day, I was steeped in a paralyzing depression, my body felt leaden, and I didn't have the energy to get out of bed. Larry was worried that I was starting another long cycle of tuning out completely and so called our family therapist, Ted, to come over. When he arrived, Ted sat on the bed next to me.

I told him about the previous day and how lonely it ended up making me feel as the reality had settled in that it was too late now to have a healthy relationship with Mother. I thought about how many mother-daughter relationships end with unresolved bereavement when the mother passes away.

Ted listened and then offered up his opinion that my depression was mainly caused by my lack of connection and ties with the women in my family. Wynonna and I rarely saw each other and there were no signs that was going to change anytime soon since she was on the road for many days each month. I missed her desperately and wondered if she thought of me. Mother, who was now in an assisted living facility, didn't seem to care if she spoke to me or if I visited.

My mother was suffering her own panic attacks, though not remotely based in reality, one night calling 911 and screaming that a Mexican cartel was there to kidnap her. She also called the fire department another night, screaming that the facility was on fire, then filled her microwave with metal objects and turned it on.

She tried to escape her new nursing home a couple of times to return to the only place she had lived for the last sixty-five years. Sadly, my younger sister and brother had sold our family home in Ashland months before. I had no chance to say goodbye to the place where I grew up. It was gone and I experienced the loss deeply, like a death in the family. All of my eccentric, mentally ill aunts had passed on, leaving me without older living relatives.

*   *   *

As 2013 came to a bitter end, I cried often throughout each day over everything that remained unresolved in my life. I wanted to call Wynonna every day, but I worried that I would drag her down emotionally while she was on tour, working so hard. I didn't trust myself to contact her without explaining that my constant daily struggles with anxiety and depression were uncontrollable and exhausting. Through therapy, I had become aware that that as my oldest child, Wy had been affected by my divorce from Michael, our early poverty, my fear of the ex-con, my struggle to support us, and our constant relocations, probably more than Ashley, because she was four years older. It frightened me that Wy might be feeling about me the way I felt about my own mother, untrusting. If that were true, I didn't know how or when our relationship would fully mend.

In my teenage years, close friends of mine would point out to me that they thought Mother was jealous of me. I scoffed at the possibility. After all, I wanted to look up to my mother. Decades later, through soul-searching and talk therapy, I had come to realize that my friends had true insight. Mother's jealousy of me, along with her resentment, had been a lifelong syndrome. I was also a "daddy's girl," and any small amount of affection that I received from him would be met with Mother's rejecting scorn for days on end. I was always emotionally perplexed by her reactions. No matter what aspect of life I excelled in—academics, popularity, style, or financially—it only met with her not-so-hidden resentment. It was difficult to accept.

The May 2015 issue of *Psychology Today* magazine contained an article that asserted a mother's jealousy is "the last dirty secret: the topic no one really wants to talk about but should." The content was based on a study that indicated that many mothers felt a boost in self-esteem if their sons achieved a lifestyle and success beyond their own, but felt worse when their daughters surpassed what they had accomplished.

When I was in high school, and throughout my show business life, Mother lived vicariously through me. If I had been invited to one of the fancy dances at the country club, she would wait up for me, drinking coffee at the kitchen table. I would have to sit down and give her every detail of who was there, what they wore, what band played, and how the country club was decorated. She never asked if I had enjoyed myself.

Later in life, I could see how Mother felt a deep inferiority, knowing she would never be invited to join the country club, for financial reasons. She had an insatiable curiosity about people in Ashland, who she perceived had a higher social status, while she simultaneously had a deep resentment and sour verbal opinion of them. Yet I know she would have given almost anything to become a member of the country club. (I was later able to buy Mother a membership, which made her happy for a few days.)

Because I was a popular teenager and had a buoyant personality, I would be invited into many different social circles. I had a great curiosity about people and was equally comfortable hanging out with the "hoods" as I was at a sock hop with the cheerleaders. I was invited to many different parties and events, and this worked in my favor at home. At first I liked the extra attention my mother gave me over these special invitations and occasions. Then I realized it wasn't out of happiness for me; it was because she wanted to hear about others and the life she thought she would never live.

In my early thirties, when the girls and I shared a dingy one-bedroom apartment in Lagunitas, California, I was putting myself through my second year of nursing school in Marin County and working in a restaurant in the evening hours. Ashley and I shared a deloused St. Vincent charity mattress on the living room floor and sleepwalking Wynonna had a twin bed in her own room. I was barely staying afloat, and relied on insurance from the state's Children and Family Services Division for my daughters and on food stamps to get by.

One day I heard an announcement at church that there was a housebound diabetic man who needed a nurse to change the bandages that covered the sores on his legs. I met with him and he offered me twenty-five dollars in cash per week to help him. That was good money to me for food and clothing for the girls, so I squeezed it into my already chaotic schedule. I remember mentioning my good fortune over the phone to Mother. I was so stressed from the long hours, going to classes, studying, helping the girls with homework, then going to my waitress job, that occasionally a coworker would take pity on me and we would share a joint to relax after our shift at the restaurant, while we wiped down all of the tables. It was the 1970s. For almost everyone I knew, smoking pot was preferred over drinking.

I never figured out how Mother found out that I occasionally smoked pot, but she thought it was her moral duty to report me to Children and Family Services. She didn't report me for smoking marijuana; she turned me in for making one hundred dollars in cash from the diabetic patient and not claiming it as income. I had to undergo an investigation and almost lost the medical benefits for my girls, her own granddaughters. This was only one of the many vengeful things my mother did that made no sense to me, until therapists helped me to understand that it was based in jealousy.

After this incident, Mother barely spoke to me for the next seven years, until the day came when there was a reversal in her attitude. Suddenly she wanted to be right by my side, running to greet me with her arms outstretched as though it was only fate that had cruelly separated us.

Chapter 13
On the Good Ship *Lollipop*

S
eeing Mother's unbridled exuberance as she burst from her front door, crossing her driveway toward our tour bus, her arms waving a warm welcome, was like watching a complete stranger. I had never seen her like this before.

She was ecstatic that I had decided to make a quick detour from our schedule, into Ashland for the night. It was the week Wynonna and I had our first write-up in *People* magazine, which in 1984 was a media event that signified a new level of fame. It was a big deal for our careers and we were proud as peacocks.

Considering that Mother had barely spoken a word to me in seven years, her manic show of happiness upon my arrival was baffling, to say the least. She was dressed up and had full makeup on. I was surprised that the local press had somehow found out about my arrival and was there with flashbulbs popping. In my deep need to have Mother's approval, I took this display as her way to let me know she was proud of me. I was so wrong.

Once out of the public eye, she didn't speak of anything besides her desire to attend our concerts and any red carpet events. This would become the template of my relationship with her and how she interacted with me. If there was a chance for her to share the spotlight, she was ready to step in at a moment's notice. The public saw her as a sweet and supportive mother, but I sadly knew otherwise.

I was happy to make her feel important, knowing that for most of her life she had no chance to have a fun or a comfortable life. She married at age fifteen, and had me when she was eighteen, and then my three younger siblings followed, each two years apart. She had no help when she brought her babies home from the hospital. Her own mother was absent from her life. Daddy didn't do any domestic chores at all. I doubt he ever changed a diaper or gave any of us a bottle. After I had Wynonna, I could more deeply empathize with the hard life my mother led. She had gone from raising her own brother and sister to taking care of Daddy and then raising children. She had no opportunity to express herself. No one asked her what would make her happy. I'm not sure she could have answered that question.

I loved Mother and wanted her to know it. But it was one-sided. She could never say "I love you" to me, unless it was a mumbled "You, too" in response to my saying it first. She has never signed a letter or even a birthday card with "Love, Mom," only "Mother."

She anticipated the chance to go on the road with us for at least part of every tour. She would glory in the moment when I would let the crowd know that my mother was in the audience. She would be sure to tell me exactly where she would be sitting so I could tell our lighting technician where to shine the spotlight. She would smile and wave as the spotlight found her, delighting in the welcoming cheers from fans.

I invited her to attend almost every awards show, mentioning her from the stage every time we won, and made sure she attended almost every red carpet event on my calendar. I would buy her a new dress, jewelry, and shoes for each occasion, have her hair and makeup done, get her a special manicure, and made certain she had an "all access" backstage pass. She was so pleasant and friendly, everyone thought she was great. No one had ever spoiled my mother, and I found a certain level of satisfaction in being able to make her finally feel special. She would grab my arm and whisper to me about which celebrities she wanted me to ask to take a photo with her. In press photos of Wy and me at any event, Mother is in most of the pictures.

At the Grammys, before the show even started she was hyperfocused on getting to meet Jack Nicholson. I only know him casually, not well, so I told Mother, "You can't do that until after the show." For the next three hours, every fifteen minutes she would ask me, "When is the show over?" I had the photo of her beaming next to Jack Nicholson enlarged and framed. She still has it displayed on her dresser in the nursing home, next to family photos.

Whenever she returned to Ashland from one of our events or tours she would have her own social spotlight for the next three or four weeks. She knew that people in small-town Ashland would want to know every detail of celebrity life. She relished being able to answer questions like, "What is Garth Brooks really like?" Or "Did you get a close look at Dolly Parton?" She would walk slowly from shop to shop downtown, being fawned over like a celebrity in her own right. For once in her life she was no longer anonymous.

It was probably the best gift I could have given Mother. She may not have had the finances to be among the elite in Ashland, but her daughter and two granddaughters were famous and that carried plenty of influence. I could appreciate her joy at this new social status, but I was constantly disappointed that she didn't seem to appreciate how hard I worked or that I wanted her to be my mother first.

One of the great benefits of the intense talk therapy I went through at Scottsdale was that it showed me how my mother's inability to validate me as a worthy daughter had warped my sense of self for decades. If looked at in a positive light, her lack of maternal warmth and encouragement was probably the strongest motivating factor for me to make something of my life.

I'm proud of the life I built for myself and especially proud of Wynonna and Ashley, their talent, intelligence, generosity, and humanitarian hearts. I try to make certain that they both know it, though I think mothers and daughters will always have a sensitivity about their interactions with each other that is more heightened than in any other relationship.

To be raised by an emotionally unavailable and unresponsive mother left me with an ever-present feeling of abandonment that is a gaping hole in my psyche. No matter how old I get, my biggest fear is being alone. I try to keep myself in check, to not let my fear of abandonment inform the way I am with my daughters, but I am not always successful. When my daughters were younger, I would tell them we were each one side of a triangle, which was only complete and strong with all three of us together. I still overreact to their fierce independence, because I don't want to lose them, but I rarely try to give them advice. Ideally, I'd like to be like a firefighter and just come when I'm called.

Shortly before I was diagnosed with hepatitis C, I was in the Northeast for a tour, followed by various events. It had been a frigid winter week and my health was taking a turn for the worse. I still had more tour dates to complete, but with a few days off I decided to rest and recover at Mother's house in Ashland. After two previous flights, I caught a hopper flight into Huntington, West Virginia, and asked Mother to pick me up at the airport. On the flight, my sore throat roared into full-blown inflammation and my head was aching. By the time the plane landed I was flat worn out, sick, and exhausted.

As I got in Mother's car I blurted out, "I'm so happy to be home. All I want is to have something to eat, take a hot bath, and then go straight to bed."

As we drove into Ashland, my mother made a turn in the opposite direction from the house.

When I asked what was going on, she announced, "I have a new manicurist, Charlotte. She really wants to meet you."

I shook my head no. "Please, Mother. I can't even smile I'm so exhausted. I'll meet her tomorrow."

She ignored my plea and drove to the salon. I could see through the window that there were eight strangers waiting to meet me. I took a minute to run a brush through my hair and apply fresh lipstick, but I still looked like a cat pulled out of a well. I dreaded having to be social, but it was obvious that I wouldn't be able to rest until I fulfilled Mother's selfish wishes, once again. After about ninety minutes of small talk and photographs with each employee and invited guest at the salon, we finally got back to the car.

Mother glowed with self-satisfaction all the way to her house. I glowed, too, from a high fever.

The next year I planned a huge birthday party for Mother. I took her to the stationery store to pick out a design for her invitations. She wanted to have about eighty guests, so I rented out the nicest restaurant in town, along with a combo of musicians to play her favorite songs. I promised I would stay next to her and sign autographs and take pictures with whoever asked, which delighted her.

All of our family, Larry, Wy, and Ashley, and my siblings and their children were in town for the event, and most of us stayed at the house. I craved one-on-one time with them to catch up on our lives. The only thing I asked of Mother was to please not let any fans or press into the house while I was staying with her. It was one of the few times I ever requested anything of Mother. I had finally set a boundary. The morning after the big party, I was coming down the stairs in my bathrobe at eight o'clock, craving a cup of strong coffee and chat time with my siblings. Through the front window I could see a man in a "Judds" ball cap sitting on the front step. He was a superfan. Before I could stop her, Mother ignored her promise to me and opened the front door, inviting him in for a cup of coffee, breakfast, an autograph, and time with me, in person. I was furious with her for stealing the precious time I had to catch up with my sister and brother and nieces and nephews and hear about their lives. I knew that if the fan was sitting at our kitchen table when they came downstairs, they would be upset, too.

I tiptoed up the stairs and packed my suitcase. I called my tour bus driver and blurted out, "Come get me. I'm out of here." I left from the back door without saying goodbye to anyone. Mom didn't have a clue about what boundaries meant.

A couple of nights later, I turned on the TV in my hotel room to see footage of my childhood bedroom and my mother describing me as a girl. She had invited *Hard Copy* into the house even though I was long gone. I guess the only lure she could promise them was a peek into the closet of my teenage years and a couple of photos long left behind in a dresser drawer. It was humiliating and I felt invaded, but I was willing to let it be the past, especially when Mother told me she had "no idea it was a tabloid TV show." When they asked what it was like raising me, she replied, "It was like having Shirley Temple in the house," rewriting my desperately unhappy childhood as her own Hollywood fantasy.

The next time one of our tours had a stop in Lexington, Kentucky, I decided to surprise Mother by leasing a coach and picking up all of her friends and neighbors to attend the concert. I loaded the bus with snacks and drinks. I told Mother she could invite whomever she wanted and they would all have free tickets in one of the first couple of rows. This was a special concert, being filmed for a CBS TV special about the Judds.

Mother became like a cruise ship director and the life of the party. During the concert, she insisted that I not only acknowledge her, but also include the names of the twenty-four people she had invited. I hesitated, thinking that the ticket-paying audience didn't care about that, but I proceeded to do what she asked, not wanting to upset her. Apparently, I left off one name as I hurriedly introduced them down the row. After the concert, when I thought my mother would be appreciative of the trouble I went to in making sure everyone had fun, she wouldn't look at me or speak to me. She was furious that I had neglected to mention the young pastor's name and title. He didn't seem to mind, but Mother sure did.

One of my favorite roadies finally approached me to inquire, "I know it's none of my business, Mamaw, but why do you let your mother treat you that way?"

I was so used to being treated disrespectfully by Mother that I forgot that other people, besides my family and friends, were noticing. It was embarrassing, but eye-opening. Still, I tilled the garden of this relationship with Mother, hoping to find a new beginning where something might have a chance of breaking through and growing.

These memories of my relationship with my mother began to surface as I tried my hardest to stay afloat, back home in Franklin. I didn't want to be hospitalized again, so I did my best to keep my anguish to myself.

I've always been good at compartmentalizing my emotions. It allowed me to do what I needed to do to survive when I was young. During my singing career, being able to compartmentalize was helpful, too, as so many people relied on my judgment and decision making for important issues. But now my emotions overflowed with each new memory and I couldn't seem to push them away unless I was distracted with something else. As soon as the sun set every night my anxiety level would rise. I would know that with the night-time would come the quiet in which my thoughts would push to the surface, refusing to be ignored. Hell was the long hours of winter darkness. I rarely slept and had begun taking Klonopin every single night, sometimes three or four within eight hours. By 3 a.m. my thoughts would carry me once again to the imagined relief of suicide.

I decided to write my will. Larry and I had already started the process before the Encore tour because I wanted to be sure our gorgeous farm that I'd worked so hard to get and the land would be protected, but now I became obsessed with having the will completed. My frame of mind was that my life could end at any minute. I mourned the person I felt had already died.

I have often said to audiences that attend my speeches that our tombstones are engraved with the date we were born and the date we die. In between the dates is the dash. The life you lead, what happens during that dash, is what is important. As a performer, I've had an electronic press kit for years, which gives the viewer a three-minute overview of my career. It was always a source of satisfaction. Now that I was certain my career was over, it seemed as if that three minutes would be all I would be remembered for.

During my panic attacks at night, since I couldn't sleep, I would clean out my drawers and closets. I started to give away my clothing, some to friends, some to charity, by the armloads. I gave away handbags and belts and most of my jewelry. I did everything with the mindset that I had very little time left.

At one point I found the small handgun I had hidden in my boot months before. I carefully held it in my hand. The metal was cool and solid. I walked into the bathroom and stared in the mirror. I held the gun up to the side of my head and looked at my face in the mirror. I thought about my grandfather, Howard. Did my maternal grandmother, Edie Mae, murder him or did he actually pull the trigger and end his own life? It suddenly didn't seem like such a terrible way to go. The gun I held wasn't loaded, but my hand trembled at the thought of what it would take to pull the trigger. Suddenly Larry appeared unexpectedly in the mirror as he came up from behind me. His eyes were filled with fear and he gently unfolded my hand from the empty gun and took it away. He couldn't even speak to me for almost an hour.

My depression and anxiety had such an effect on Larry that he had gone into his own tailspin since my return from Scottsdale. He had also been prescribed Klonopin by his general practitioner to help him deal with the stress at home. He soon figured out that I was sneaking pills from his prescription, which is how he knew I was back on it myself.

When he could talk, he said one thing: "I'm not going to leave you alone at all, anymore. Not until you get better." And he didn't. I was under constant observation every waking moment.

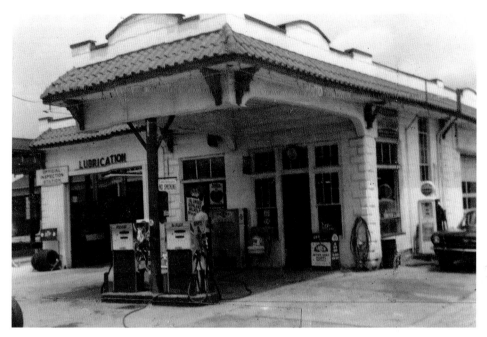

ABOVE: I would walk two blocks over to Daddy's station just to be around him. BELOW: My brothers (left to right) Brian, before he got sick, and Mark, who is clowning around, on a summer afternoon with Mother and Daddy.

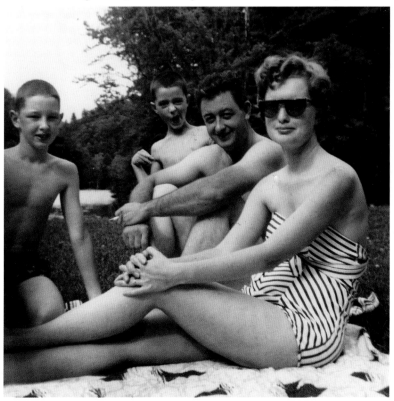

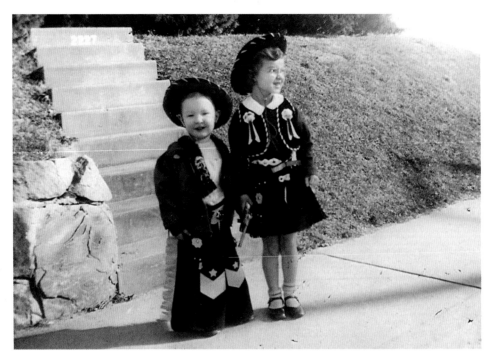

ABOVE: Brian and I were best buddies; we were always together. BELOW: Pets have always been my great love. Here I am with my brothers and our first dog, Duchess, at the farm.

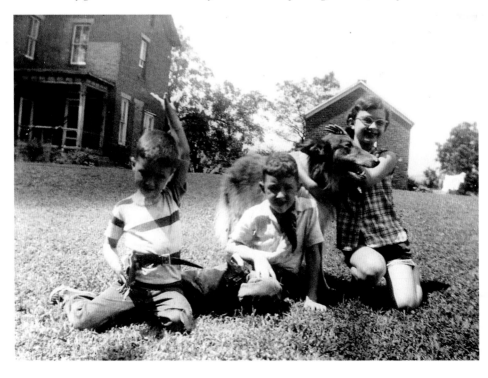

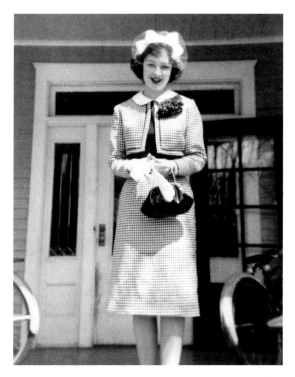

ABOVE: I was very prim and proper. I played piano at the Baptist church on Sunday mornings.
BELOW: We moved to Nashville in 1979 and I worked as an RN while my girls were in school.

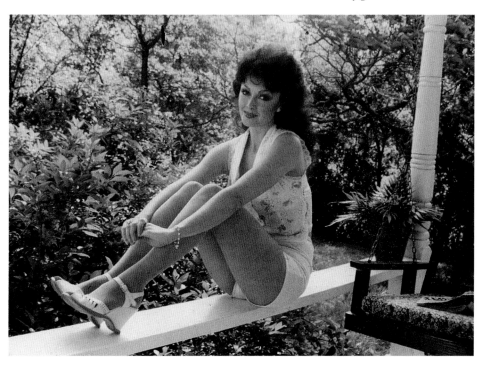

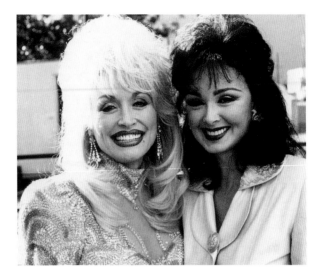

ABOVE: I am so proud to call Dolly my friend. She's the most brilliant woman I've ever known.

BELOW: With my lovely daughters in 1984. Notice the Maytag wringer washer on the back porch.

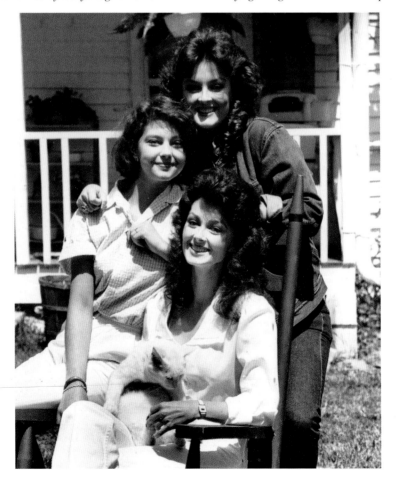

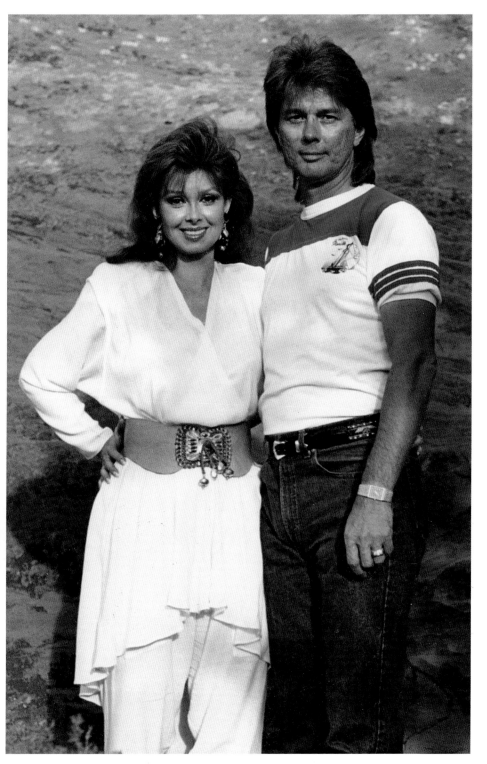

Larry told me he was madly in love with me on our third date.

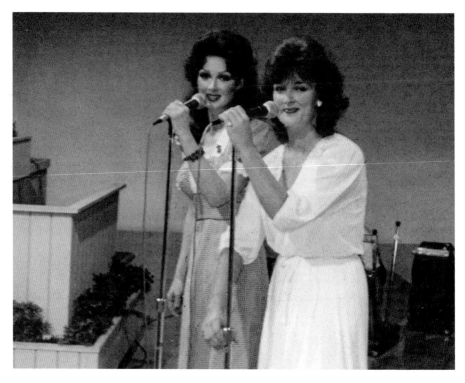

Above: Our first live TV performance in 1982, at 5 a.m. on a local TV show. Wy was eighteen when we started singing.

Below: When I travel for a speaking gig, I love to spend time hanging out with those in the medical profession.

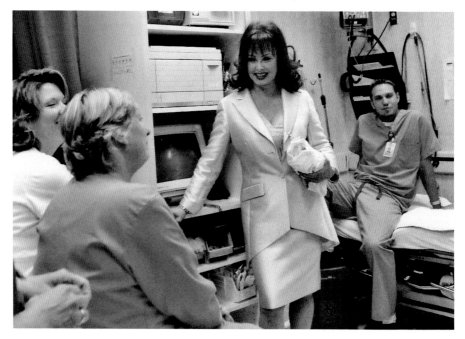

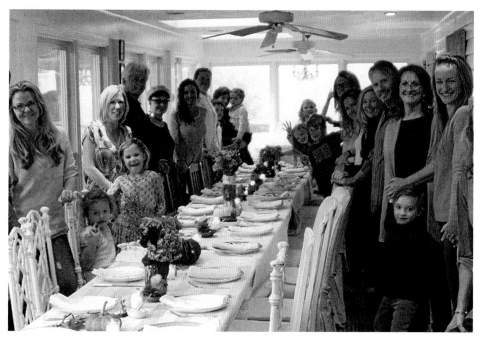

Above: The multi-generations that gather for our "family of choice" Sunday get-togethers keep Larry and me feeling young.

Below: Poet, novelist, civil rights activist, and Presidential Medal of Freedom recipient, Maya Angelou, slicing into the pineapple upside down cake I made for her.

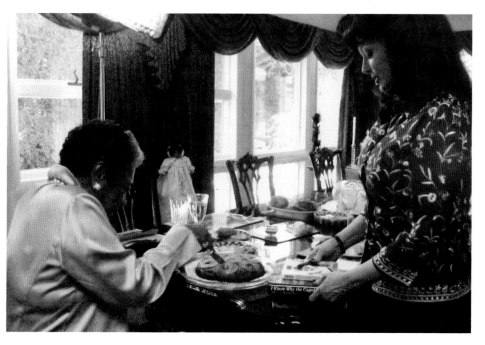

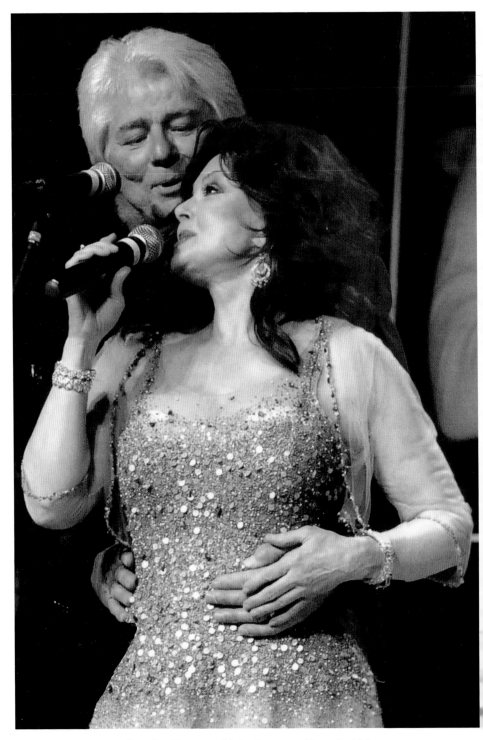

*Sometimes Larry would sing harmony with me. I wish I
had known him when he was singing backup for Elvis.*

Chapter 14

May I Borrow Your Hammer?

r. Mona Lisa Schulz and I had been talking by phone at least once a week since my return from Scottsdale. She could tell by my voice and reaction to her questions that I was slipping lower and lower. I didn't tell her that I had self-prescribed Klonopin from my hidden stash and even had asked my general practitioner doctor to write a prescription for more, which he gave me without asking questions. I didn't tell her but it's hard to hide something from such a gifted medical intuitive, so Dr. Mona Lisa already knew. It's uncanny being around her, since she knows things about you before you can tell her.

She convened a family meeting with Larry and Ashley once again.

The truth came spilling out that I was taking Klonopin again. I was very forthright that I refused to go through the risky phenobarbital detox protocol at Vanderbilt a second time.

Dr. Mona Lisa already had an alternate idea. She felt strongly that I needed treatment specifically for my panic disorder, because that was what had pushed me back toward Klonopin. Her suggestion was inpatient therapy at a rehabilitation facility in Malibu, California. This would have three benefits: get me through Klonopin withdrawal, teach me coping skills to deal with panic attacks, and be in sunny California during the winter. Everyone was in agreement that this was a good idea, except for me. The thought of being in another situation where I would be under observation twenty-four hours a day, treated like a child, and have my days and nights structured and monitored made me want to kick and scream like a toddler being forced to an early bedtime. I did not want to go.

Larry wouldn't be able to stay with me, but he vowed to find a nearby hotel to live in and promised to be with me for every available visiting hour. I still dreaded having to go, but I was more concerned that Larry would give up on me if I didn't go. He couldn't keep up his currently imposed arrangement of never leaving me alone. He was trapped in the house with me and I was feeling completely mistrusted. I knew he had every reason to not trust what I would do next, because I doubted my own ability to reason in reality.

Singer Stevie Nicks has been very public about how difficult it is to detox from benzodiazepines like Klonopin. After Stevie went through rehabilitation for an addiction to cocaine in the late 1980s, she was prescribed Klonopin. She went on it and didn't get off for eight years.

When I met Stevie more than a decade ago, she described the feeling of her addiction to me, but at that time I could only sympathize, because I didn't have an addiction issue. She told me that her creativity vanished on Klonopin. She felt calm but completely dead inside. She said she became a "whatever" person who didn't care about anything anymore.

Remembering this conversation with Stevie Nicks made me shudder in anticipation of what I could become. I've never been known as a woman without passion or drive. Having a cause or a purpose has always mattered greatly to me. I took Stevie's warning words as a harbinger of my future if I continued taking Klonopin.

Yet her description of the detox process scared me equally. I hoped that it wouldn't be as severe as Stevie described: "My hair turned gray. My skin molted. I couldn't sleep; I was in so much pain. Legs aching, muscle cramps . . . The rock star in me wanted to get in a limousine and go to Cedars-Sinai and say, 'Give me some Demerol because I am in pain.' And the other side of me said, 'You will fight out this forty-seven days.' I felt like somebody opened up a door and pushed me into hell."

The rehab treatment facility in Malibu, Promises, is in a lovely, expansive resort-type of building with large sun-filled windows, set far back into the hillside from the main road. There is nothing that looks threatening or institutional about this place. Still, I was feeling like I was rushing headlong into "hell."

When Larry drove me up the long private road to the treatment facility, his face reflected both somber resignation and relief that the end of my problems might be in sight. I could feel my heart thumping against my rib cage and my hands were tingling and turning numb. It was difficult to take a deep breath in. I realized that being able to take a Klonopin when I thought I needed one would no longer be an option. This terrified me since I had become very dependent on it, once again, in the last four months. I knew as I was admitted for this inpatient treatment that everything would be taken away. In preparation, I thought I was being crafty and hid a couple of Klonopin in the strap of my bra. I wanted to have them available, just in case it got really bad. It didn't work. Promises is pretty used to desperate clients trying to come prepared. They go through everything you bring with you, including the clothing on your body. I found the search invasive and humiliating. I wondered what would it take to convince Larry to take me back home.

*   *   *

Everything visual about Promises would make you think you were there on vacation, from the beautiful landscaping to the spa and swimming pool; a massage therapist and acupuncturist were there almost daily. However, you aren't there for fun or good memories. From the first day it becomes very clear that your schedule is not your own. In many aspects it's like being locked up in a high-end jail. Almost every waking hour is scheduled and even during your free time you are still under observation. This would be my life for at least the next month. I begged Larry to not leave me there. He gently reminded me that nothing else had worked thus far.

The curriculum at PCS in Scottsdale had many hours of individual therapy with the adage, "If you can't name it, you can't solve it." In Malibu, it was the complete opposite. Twice daily patients would all meet in one large room for therapy called "Process Group." Often these ninety-minute sessions had outside speakers, professionals who would lecture about specific topics like skills to prevent a relapse into alcohol or drug use. The group sessions seemed endless, since most of the information the speaker was giving was not new to me. I am well-read on many psychological techniques so I would get extremely bored as the speakers droned on. Plus, I actually speak on these topics myself. My fuse was pretty short, especially as I was detoxing from Klonopin. I was restless and resented having to be there at all and I let everyone know it, too. I had no filter left between my thoughts and my speech.

One afternoon a dull-as-dirt psychologist who was robotically talking about the eight stages of psychosocial development, from Erik Erikson's model, noticed I was jiggling my foot with impatience, which he must have thought was rude. With a snippy tone, he asked me if I knew the names of the eight stages.

Of course I do, I replied. I took a deep breath, like I do when I have to sing a particularly long phrase. "Trust versus Mistrust. Stage One. Stage Two is Autonomy versus Shame and Doubt." I rattled them off before he cut me off with, "Well, if you know so much, why are you here?"

I could tell that he was purposely trying to shame me in front of the group. I wasn't having it.

"I'm here because I have a disease of my brain," I snapped and then added, "but I can see exactly what your problem is, you fat-ass moron." The other patients started to laugh. The frustrated therapist was now angry and declared that he was going to report my behavior.

I stood up and yelled, "Go ahead. You have borderline personality disorder with impotence problems!" His hands were balled into fists at his sides and I thought momentarily that he might come after me. The only response I felt was: Finally! Some excitement!

The room fell silent. Everyone looked at me as though Toto had pulled the curtain open revealing that the Wizard of Oz was a dumpy psychologist going through the motions of doing his job. Were we really afraid of him "reporting" us? Did we have to endure speakers who wanted to be there less than we did? One of the other patients raised his hand and said, "We'd like Naomi to lead the group from now on. We like her better, plus she knows more."

The others clapped and whistled in agreement. I didn't intend to rouse the rebels, but it reminded me that I have a strong mind of my own, a mind that would hopefully heal and return me to the woman I once was.

To pass the time, I found myself observing the personalities of my fellow patients at Promises, the eleven other people in my group.

We became a tribe. The Mamaw Judd side of my personality asserted itself as I questioned each person about his or her life and spent time dispensing comfort or courage. It was helpful to both of us.

One twenty-something woman was admitted for her second stay after a relapse on drugs. I could tell she felt strangely at home and protected in this setting. I discovered that her parents were wealthy globe-trotters who were happy to pay for her treatment instead of participating in her therapy. Promises became like family to her. I thought she probably would not make it past her addiction if there weren't more acceptance and love for this girl in the real world.

Another patient was the son of a well-known politician and had gotten into the habit of drinking red wine and taking Klonopin to relax. He never expected to lose control over his ability to get by without it, but finally he had to admit he was powerless to change his habit. Larry and I would spend our visitations with him. There was too much potential for scandal or tabloid leaks if his parents visited and people saw him with his famous family.

One of the most famous singers in the world was there, as well as a woman who looked like a June Cleaver–style housewife. You would never pick her out in a crowd for having a heroin problem. The insidious nature of addiction floods across every social, racial, educational, and economic line. More than 20 million people in the United States have an addiction problem; that's one in ten Americans. People who are depressed are more likely to have an addiction problem.

A week after I arrived, a young man from New York City checked in. He was slender, well dressed, and wore black horn-rimmed glasses. He was given a room directly across from mine. He seemed paranoid and high-strung and after I gave him a hug of welcome on the first day, he began to shadow me everywhere I went for the next week. He would save me a seat at every group session and would come into my room uninvited.

I tried to keep my distance from him since I had a strong intuitive feeling that there was much more to his story than depression or anxiety.

Every resident was allowed two and a half hours of free time on Saturday nights to leave the premises. It was the only time I felt a semblance of being myself again. Larry would pick me up and we'd drive into Santa Monica. I'd sit close to him and we'd sing along with the radio. We would always go to the famous restaurant, the Ivy at the Shore. I've been dozens of times and could call the waiters by name. Being near the ocean was restorative and eating dinner in a restaurant full of happy locals or vacationers reminded me that the real world was still happening outside my own personal turmoil. I wanted to be done with rehabilitation, and would plead for Larry to drive me back to Tennessee. Every time he visited me at Promises or dropped me off after our Saturday date, he would have tears in his eyes. If I wasn't motivated to get better for myself, I certainly wanted to recover for the love of my life.

There was a curfew on Saturday nights, and as soon as you returned you had to give a urine sample and blow into a Breathalyzer as proof that you had not cheated. I felt like a criminal. On the second Saturday, the young man from New York returned on time but got into trouble when he offered a sum of money and begged one of the other clients to take his urine test for him because he was drunk. The "testing" room was very close to my bedroom and I could overhear every word of his escalating argument that he was being treated unfairly.

There were no internal locks on any of the rooms and I was feeling unsafe and on edge and expressed my concern to the staff.

I noticed right away that they couldn't reassure me that everything was fine. In fact, they seemed harried and distracted. Suddenly, out of nowhere, police cars came ripping up the driveway with sirens wailing and lights flashing.

I hollered to everyone, who were startled by the appearance of law enforcement, "I bet I know who they're here to get. Come on! We need to get to the front windows."

Minutes later we saw the police quickly escort the belligerent young man from New York City out of the building in handcuffs and shove him in the back of a squad car.

Of course, it was a mystery I couldn't leave unsolved. One of the techs informed me that the young man had bludgeoned his psychiatrist to death in New York with a hammer the previous month and had flown to Los Angeles hoping to hide in the rehab facility. He was on the FBI's "Most Wanted" list. And this violent murderer had been in the room directly across from mine! I had hugged him and put up with his weirdness. This made me look around the room at the rest of the clients and wonder what their secrets were.

Almost every night, as I got ready for bed, I would feel increasing fear about having another panic attack. Nighttime was when it seemed almost impossible to quiet my frantic mind. To each worry I had I would attach the worst-case scenario of an outcome. My mind would replay the threat over and over. If I managed to fall asleep, I would often awaken with a feeling of dread from some past toxic memory that was once again creeping to the surface. If there was no specific memory, the thought of "Will I suffer from this for the rest of my life?" was enough to provoke a full-on panic attack. I longed to be home, where I could pace the hallways until morning.

*   *   *

Promises was the first place to give me the practical skills to deal with my panic attacks. I met with a therapist who specialized in panic disorder. She told me that the most important thing to remember is that the panic attack will pass. It was important to feel the fear and then remind myself that I would not die. No one has died from a panic attack, though it feels like you might. One in three people who go to the emergency room thinking they are having a heart attack are actually having a panic attack.

The therapist even taught me about the neuroscience of a panic attack. The limbic system of the body is overactive, causing the amygdala to go into "fight or flight" mode. The amygdala was one of the first parts of the primitive human brain to develop and had great importance when man had to outrun a charging animal out to kill. It's located deep in the brain's temporal lobes. Even though we rarely have to outrun a ravenous bear coming out of hibernation, the amygdala has a default operation that can kick in for things that are not life threatening, such as a verbal argument or an emotional memory of a difficult time. I was taught that the best way to get through a panic attack was to convince my hypersensitive limbic mind that it was fine. One method was to force myself into the current moment by noticing my surroundings.

When I could feel a panic attack mounting inside me, I was encouraged to practice a deep breathing technique and channel my mind into focusing on something completely mundane that kept me busy in the present moment, such as counting the slats in the window blinds, and then counting the tiles in the floor at my feet. I could notice the colors in the art on the wall. Guess how many inches the chair was from the bed. I was to focus on any material thing that would keep my mind in the here and now. If I woke up with a panic attack, I was to remain in bed until it passed; I was advised that this would train my mind to believe I was safe.

At Promises, they try to replace your dependency on a strong drug, like Klonopin, with safe and effective nonaddictive medications that help the withdrawal process to be less painful. Still, the replacement drugs have far less potency and it was very noticeable for someone like me, who had been taking three or four Klonopin to make it through a night. I had become hooked on it over the past four months and the withdrawal symptoms were severe. My anxiety increased, my leg and arm muscles felt constantly clenched in spasms, and I had an omnipresent headache and nightly insomnia. If I was lucky enough to fall asleep, the nightmares would soon have me awake and jumping out of bed, my heart racing.

The sleeping medication given to me was mild and would only help me to feel a bit more relaxed, but not at all sleepy. After three sleepless nights in a row, I felt desperate to have a night of rest. I discussed this with the RNs who oversaw the medications, but they were unwilling to up the dosage. The next day, out of sheer desperation, I devised my own plan.

I had made friends with a nighttime staff person, a young, impressionable man with a great sense of humor who could be easily embarrassed. I had chosen him for my scheme. He would dispense medications from his small desk each night, as I sat next to him. He would lay my medications out on the desk as a way to count them and then put them into a container. I wore a bathrobe into the medication room to pick up my nightly distribution and tucked my hands in the pockets. On my left hand, I rolled up a piece of Scotch tape across my palm. I waited until he had laid out a number of medications and then surprised him with this question: "So exactly how big is your penis?"

His eyes opened wide in surprise and then he tipped his head back to laugh. In that split second, I placed my hand, palm down, on the desk and the tape picked up five pills in one quick motion. When he was done laughing, he wiped his eyes and tried to continue counting pills. I could see that he had been thrown off in the process of dispensing. He would have to start over.

That night I was able to take two sleeping pills, instead of the one prescribed. I was finally able to sleep for six hours in a row. It was heaven. The pull of finding relief through taking another pill is so strong with addiction that you set aside any moral conflict, thinking that you're not hurting anyone else. My scheme worked perfectly—until one of the nurses entered my room unexpectedly and caught me counting the pills I had scored the night before.

"Oh my goodness," the nurse gasped. "What do you have here?" She moved me aside and swept the pills into her hand and took them away. Then she searched the rest of my room for hidden pills. Later that day, she put out a bulletin to the other staff members that I wasn't to be trusted. It hurt my feelings, even though my actions deserved the alert notice. I had earlier bonded with this nurse over our similar experiences working in emergency rooms. Now the bond was broken and my nights of good sleep would be over, too.

She looked at me the next day and asked, "Do you want to get better or not? We're here for you. But it's your choice."

At that time it didn't feel like my choice. When you're depressed you feel debilitated. Your judgment is off because your mind is in distress, which short-circuits your ability to reason. I would have surges of motivation to get better for Larry and my girls, but soon the hopeful feelings would be blotted out with a black cloud of despair. I looked at everything that was happening through a negative filter because my ability to see the bigger picture was warped. I wasn't certain how I would live to see the next week.

At the end of my third week at Promises, I was irritable and feeling caged in. The therapists were already suggesting that I stay for additional time, as they were concerned I would find a way to go back on Klonopin to deal with my chronic anxiety. It seemed like all my energy was going into trying to control myself, instead of recovering and going home.

One night, as I lay in bed, I could feel my heart starting to pound in a frighteningly fast rhythm. I tried sitting on the edge of my bed and counting the tiles across the edge of the floor, but soon my eyesight blurred and I felt dizzy. One of the nurses tried to calm me down and talk me through it, but I was convinced I would never be able to catch my breath, as I couldn't seem to inhale deeply at all. The nurse conferred with other staff members and decided to call Larry at his hotel. They advised him to take me to the emergency room at UCLA Medical Center, since an hour had passed and my symptoms had not subsided.

Larry and another staff member supported me between them as I stumbled toward the car. My breathing slowed somewhat as we drove along the coast into Santa Monica, but my heart was still pounding. Once in the emergency room, I began to cry from fear and humiliation. The female doctor was very sympathetic and assured me I wasn't the first person to come into the ER in a full-fledged panic attack. She also informed that I was the third patient to come to the hospital that evening fearing they were having a heart attack when they were actually experiencing panic. She ordered a strong shot of Ativan, which is also a benzodiazepine like Klonopin, only not as long lasting. It was enough to take the edge off the panic and I could finally feel like I could cope. Ironically, before I left, the doctor wrote me a prescription for my anxiety and had it filled at the hospital pharmacy. When I got in the car with Larry, I opened the small white bag to see what I had been given. It was a packet of Klonopin. Larry shook his head and gently took the bag from my hand and tucked it into his pocket.

I was in a sleepless, dazed state all the next day, through the group therapies and my individual therapy. I didn't want to be around people at all and craved the privacy of my own home and the safety of my cozy kitchen couch. My happier life as a wife, mother, and a performer seemed like a faraway dream, one I had never lived. I couldn't concentrate on the smallest task. When Larry came to visit in the late afternoon, I sat motionless in a lawn chair in the sun as he did his best to cheer me up. His faith in my ability to recover was the one thread to which I desperately clung, though I feared seeing that committed faith missing from his eyes one day. There is more than a modicum of comfort in knowing that someone keeps praying for you, even when your own faith has collapsed under the weight of months and months of depressive darkness and emotional pain.

That night, expecting to be able to fall asleep from sheer exhaustion, I had what I would call the "grand mal" of panic attacks. It hit me like being electrocuted. I broke out in a drenching sweat from my scalp to my toes. My heart raced at such a high speed I was certain it would create an aneurysm. I wasn't able to form words and when I tried to stand up to walk, my knees wouldn't let me. My muscles twitched and jerked. I couldn't catch my breath and began to hyperventilate. This time the staff didn't try to calm me down; they summoned 911 paramedics immediately.

We raced down the driveway of Promises with lights and siren blaring. The paramedic who had transferred me to the gurney recognized me. I felt so ashamed and out of control. In the back of the ambulance, the EMT looked down at me with pity in his eyes and to assure me whispered, "Don't worry. We're going to take good care of you. You're going to be okay."

The emergency room doctor went through the necessary protocol while I lay on the narrow bed with my teeth still chattering and my heart racing. When Larry arrived, I held on to his shirtsleeve and told him I was sure I was going crazy and that I didn't think I could take it anymore. The doctor must have overheard what I said, because he convened with his staff and came back with the decision that Larry shouldn't drive me back to Malibu. They must have interpreted my thoughts as a suicidal threat. The doctor administered a shot of Ativan, the same as the night before, but this time added a dose of Seroquel. I have no memory of the next ten hours. I wish I had no memory of the next ten days in the UCLA psych ward.

Chapter 15

When You Live in
a Glass House

My car had ended up in a deep ditch. I had lost control over it driving to attend my first day of nurse's training at Eastern Kentucky University. It was a brisk January morning when the accident happened. I had seen Wy and Ashley off on their school bus and now I was on my way to further my own education. I was elated to finally be pursuing a lifelong passion and a career I knew would support a whole new lifestyle for my daughters and me.

Halfway down the steep hill from where we lived in a tiny, unheated fishing cabin, a freak snowstorm began pummeling the windshield of my old car. I slowed to a crawl, being careful not to make any sudden moves with the steering wheel, but still my tires started skidding across the newly formed black ice. Everything went into slow motion as my huge raft of a car first slid sideways to the right, then backward, and then veered in the opposite direction across the road before sailing into the ditch and tipping over onto its side.

The force propelled me with a bruising thud onto the passenger door, flat on my back. It only took a few minutes for the blizzard to completely cover my car. Standing on the passenger door, I used all the strength I had to push open the driver's side door and crawl out. I screamed for help, but the dense snow falling all around me muffled my cry. I would have to find help on my own, because no one knew where I was and no one cared, either.

This was the memory dream I was having when I first came to consciousness in the psychiatric ward at UCLA Medical Center. When the accident had actually occurred thirty-five years before, I didn't perish in the storm. I took action, trudging through six inches of snow across a farmer's field and persuading him to tow me from the ditch with his tractor. He was busy and reluctant to help, but I used my power of persuasion topped off with some charm, and soon the giant-wheeled tractor yanked my old car back on to the road. I still made it to my first day of class. Nothing could stop me then. My fighting spirit had pulled me through thirty-six years of emotional and financial challenges. Where was that spirit now?

When I awoke in a barren room, I struggled to keep my eyes open, to distinguish the dream from a harsh new reality. It all felt like slow motion again. I only had a vague recollection of being brought here on a gurney and then transferred to this sterile-looking room. The bed I lay on with side rails and one small dresser were the only objects in the room. I noticed that the rails on the bed had holes in them, probably for tying down an out-of-control patient.

I felt like a fragile figurine in a terrarium because all four walls of my room were reinforced-glass windows. This is the type of room given to new patients so that they can be constantly observed from the nurses' station and the hallways.

This is it, I thought. I have finally been committed as an insane person to a mental ward, thousands of miles from home, in an institution where I don't know a soul. This is my real-life *One Flew Over the Cuckoo's Nest,* no longer an amusing thought, as it was while in the group at Promises. Now I really was locked up.

I was suddenly overwhelmed by a sense of powerlessness and desperation at the thought of being involuntarily held in a psychiatric ward. I could feel a whale of a panic attack mounting as my heart rate increased. I weakly called out Larry's name, praying he was there, just out of my line of vision. He wasn't. I forced myself to breathe more deeply and tried to find something to count, as suggested by the therapist at Promises. I looked for window blinds, but there were none. There was no art on the walls, not even a hook for hanging a bathrobe.

Instead of finding an object to focus on, my attention was caught by a woman with wiry unkempt hair who was pacing in front of my window, brushing against the glass like a tiger in a zoo, her hollow and lifeless eyes locked on me as if she were sizing up her prey. I wanted to get up and find a bathroom, but I didn't dare. I had no idea if this feral-appearing woman could burst through the door and attack me.

After what seemed like an hour, a nurse came in to check on me. She brought basic toiletries: a toothbrush, a plastic cup, and a small towel.

I did my best to keep my voice calm as I cautiously questioned her: "Have I been locked up?"

She answered that I hadn't been committed, but I was admitted for intense observation because they thought I was very sick with panic disorder and severe depression. She checked my vital signs, drew blood, and gave me a pair of socks to wear on my feet. Anything with strings, like shoes or drawstring sweatpants, was not allowed. For now I had only generic hospital scrubs to replace my emergency room gown and the pair of socks. It was incredibly demeaning.

After she left, a tech wheeled in a tray containing some breakfast and stayed to watch me eat it. I could barely swallow a thing, but I didn't want to appear defiant in any way. I was terrified that I would be put somewhere even worse. I couldn't imagine where that would be, considering what was happening all around me.

The noise level, even sequestered away in my observation room, couldn't be ignored. There was the loud sound of double sets of electronically locked and alarmed doors being buzzed open for staff and visitors, then clanging shut. Carts rattled through the hallways. I could hear patients yelling out incoherent things.

One young woman talked endlessly to anyone who would listen about how her parents were going to show up at any minute to kill her. She was frantic. The other patient, who was still pacing and brushing against the window of my room, started knocking on the glass to get my attention. I could hear a TV blaring from nearby. I could see two catatonic-looking patients mindlessly rocking back and forth in chairs by the nurses' station. Some man howled like a wolf at random times. I couldn't see where he was and it was nerve-racking.

The most disconcerting aspect was being under intense observation around the clock. If I was left alone, it was only for fifteen minutes at a time, before another medical technician would appear with a clipboard and silently watch me for twenty or thirty seconds and then make notes as if I were a science experiment. There was no privacy for the first seventy-two hours, even in the bathroom.

I was informed by one of the staff members that my days would be completely structured from sunup until bedtime. He encouraged me to participate in group therapy sessions that would be happening that afternoon, but I was terrified to leave the protection of my room.

When I asked if I could call my husband, they told me that Larry would only be able to visit me briefly every afternoon and not without supervision. When he was finally able to see me, hours later, it was obvious he was also terrified. He had never seen me in such a vulnerable state before and I could tell that he was trying to be careful about what he said to the nurses or staff. He didn't want to make things worse.

He worried about the state of mind of the other patients who were locked in this hospital wing with me and was afraid for my physical safety. We were both certain that I would be released as soon as a psychiatrist met with me the following morning and realized I would not be any harm to others or myself. That's not what happened.

All of my previous medications had been halted and I was put on Seroquel. I tried to gently protest, saying that it made me feel like I couldn't think or move. I explained that it had taken me weeks to get over the effects of the Seroquel I had been given at Vanderbilt. The nurse wrote something down in my chart without responding. It was then that I realized that they could interpret anything I said or did in any way they wanted and it would become a permanent statement in my chart. The slightest protest might be seen as pathology, instead of a question about how I was being medicated. I decided to keep my mouth shut. When they gave me my pill, I only swallowed half of it, hiding the other half in the runner of the dresser drawer. I knew I couldn't afford to be incoherent if I hoped to be discharged. I had to be able to speak whole sentences.

The next morning and every single morning following, I had to meet with a psychiatrist for evaluation. Much of that time was spent with me repeating and repeating my story of the treatments prior to being placed at UCLA. I was asked the same set of questions almost every morning, usually including whether I was having suicidal thoughts.

I was very careful at all times about how I responded to both the nurses and the psychiatrist. I became highly paranoid and started planning out everything I would say. I said only what I thought they wanted to hear. I was petrified that with any wrong word they would write a permanent notation on my chart to the effect that I was certifiably insane and a danger to society and myself. I imagined being locked away forever.

Joining other patients for afternoon group therapy sessions was even more of a problem for me. Many of the others seemed to be there because of a psychotic break. They were tiptoeing around the edges of reality with a delusional or distorted view. I had such a fear of having my own psychotic break that to observe these other patients created unbridled anxiety in me. It was tough to listen to some of them ramble on pointlessly.

Occasionally, there would be an outbreak of heightened emotions and escalated physicality. I steered clear as much as I could. I wanted to shout, "Get me away from these crazies," but I feared that my own emotions would be judged as hostile and aggressive and cause for more medication or even restraints. I kept my mouth firmly closed.

When I wasn't in group therapy, I would spend the rest of my time in bed. I didn't sit in the dayroom or watch TV. I didn't want to be involved with the other patients. If one of the patients tried to get into my personal space, I got silently defensive. I wasn't about to call attention to myself in a negative way, but I also wasn't going to suffer any fool who decided to mess with me.

When the frantic woman who talked endlessly about how her parents were ruining her life followed me into my room, I didn't call for help. I spun on my heels and drew back my fist, aiming for her face. I so wanted to break her jaw. She saw that I wasn't going to mess around and hightailed it down the hall. When you live in a glass room, you can't throw stones, but I sure as hell would throw a punch without regret.

Other patients on my floor seemed to be recovering from addiction issues, like me. I could intuitively tell which patients had been in a "revolving door" relationship with this psychiatric unit by their comfort in an attitude of defeat. I would have done anything to stay away after this experience, but two things became crystal clear to me in my observations of the other patients: Addiction is a powerful force and some people can only find "control" by giving up their free will to something or someone else's control. Either drugs dictated their every move or the staff in a locked psych unit did. I don't think there's an ounce of that trait in me, which is why I desperately wanted out.

When Larry would come to visit me for the brief time allowed, he would bring in food from a restaurant, so I wouldn't have to eat hospital food. I whispered to him each day when he had to leave, "Please find a way to get me discharged."

I had used the word *brokenhearted* many times in my life, but I never felt the physicality of a broken heart until I was in this psychiatric unit, with no visitors besides Larry. I didn't want my daughters to know where I was and Larry had agreed not to tell them, but I missed them both horribly. My heart hurt knowing that Wynonna and I had miles of misunderstanding now between us, which remained unresolved. Mother had asked no questions as to where I was.

When I lived in Los Angeles, Nancy, my neighbor and friend who would babysit my girls, and I had built a fun-loving "fractured family" life that worked well. She had her one little girl, Gabrielle, who was Ashley's age. We took our kids to the beach, the parks, and for walks through Beverly Hills to window-shop, anything that was free. We cooked together and would save our money for a field trip with our girls. Life was tough, but we were scrappy and undefeatable. As I remembered those hungry years, I knew I was currently starved for a feeling of connection. I had kept in touch, especially with Gabrielle, over the years, sending her gifts for her special occasions as she grew up. On a prior phone call, Gabrielle had let me know that her mom was battling cancer. I wanted to talk to Nancy, once more, about our memories and get her perspective on our lives in Los Angeles. I wrote a long letter, explaining the downward spiral of my last two years. As the days passed, it became obvious that Nancy was not well, and then Larry had heard from Gabrielle that her mother had died while I was in the psych ward. My heart ached with sadness. Nancy was one of the strongest women I knew, but her insidious disease took her life. Would my brain disease eventually take mine?

One afternoon, I decided not to attend group therapy. It was always voluntary, but the therapists and staff strongly "urged" participation. I was afraid that my not going would seem noncompliant, but I was feeling so low I couldn't face the group. For about five minutes, I stood in the hallway contemplating pushing open the door to the ward and running, even though the alarm system would sound. I wanted nothing more than to be free.

I lay on my bed and thought about my life before depression and anxiety took me prisoner. I remembered how I handled the patients who were under my care during my years working as a nurse. I was the nurse who was known for being able to calm any patient who was frightened, couldn't sleep, or might be traumatized by what might lay ahead for them. I had a good reputation for caring for their emotional needs. You know how they say someone needs "a good talking to." I've always believed the opposite: They need a good listening to.

One of my patients was a woman who had been prepped to have a pretty radical and urgent heart surgery. As the nurses came to wheel her down to surgery, the woman started yelling, "No, no, no!" Her family stood by her bedside, helpless to know what to do. The woman had changed her mind and wasn't going to go through with the operation. Her charge nurse came and found me, saying, "She needs this surgery and has to go down *now!*"

I went into her room and asked her family to please leave the two of us alone for a while. I drew the curtain around her bed for privacy. I asked her if she wanted to pray together and for the first time that day she said, "Yes." I quoted her a Bible verse, Isaiah 26:3: "Thou wilt keep him in perfect peace, whose mind is stayed on thee: because he trusted in thee." After a short prayer for peace of mind, she asked me if I thought she should have the surgery. I told her, "Honey, I would not be here if I wasn't one hundred percent sure you will be okay."

Her family was both astonished and relieved that in such a short time their loved one allowed herself to be wheeled away for the necessary surgery. I wished there were a nurse who could calm my heart in the same manner now and tell me that she was 100 percent sure I would be well again.

Almost as if a prayer had been said on my behalf, a nurse, assigned to work with me, appeared. She knew who I was and confessed that she was a longtime fan and knew the words to all of the Judds' songs. She talked to me person to person, as though we were at a meet-and-greet after a concert. She didn't make notes on her clipboard or ask me the same string of questions the other staff members did every morning and evening.

This nurse acknowledged that I was going through a bad time in life, but said it would pass and I would be myself again one day soon. She had read my chart and knew my medical history. She remarked that it was no wonder I was going through this, in light of the amount of my past trauma, which was finally catching up with me. She reminded me of all the people I had helped over the years and said that now was the time for me to pay attention to myself. On one of my worst days of doubting my sanity, she rescued me. I told her that I doubted my sanity more and more as each day passed.

The next morning she went to extraordinary lengths to help me change my perspective. I didn't know what she was up to, but I went along with her when she showed up in my room with a shopping bag stuffed with a costume for me wear.

She unfolded an extra lab coat and helped me put it on. She had brought a newsboy cap to put on my head and oversize sunglasses. From the bottom of the bag she pulled out an extra pair of tennis shoes that she kept in her locker. I had not had shoes on my feet for so long that they felt to me like I was floating on a cloud. Then she walked me out, through the two sets of locked doors that separated me from the real world.

We strolled the campus from end to end on the green grass. I inhaled the fresh air deeply and turned my face into the warm sunshine and sobbed. I was out free, in the natural world!

We chatted about everything except my being hospitalized. I even laughed once or twice. No one walking by gave me even a second look. No one was judging me. I was just another person, crossing a bustling campus on a busy day. As we circled back around to the psychiatric ward I started to cry. It wasn't out of fear of returning. I was just so thankful for this nurse's kindness and for treating me like a normal woman, if only for an hour. She gave me that gift. I believe there are angels among us, and she is one.

Behind the scenes, Larry was in daily contact with Dr. Mona Lisa, by phone, updating her on my situation. Without my knowing it, she contacted Dr. Jerrold Rosenbaum, the head of the Department of Psychiatry at Massachusetts General Hospital in Boston, the number one department in the United States for eighteen of the last twenty-one years.

She called Dr. Rosenbaum and asked him, without identifying who I was, "Can you take a look at my girlfriend's chart? She's in the UCLA psych unit and I don't think it's good for her. She's getting more despondent every day."

She asked him for a favor saying that confidentiality would be of great importance as I was a public person. He agreed to review my history and then advise her on how to get me the help I needed. Feeling hopeful and trusting of Dr. Rosenbaum's expertise, Dr. Mona Lisa reached out to Larry to have him send my chart directly to Dr. Rosenbaum. After reading my records Dr. Rosenbaum called Dr. Mona Lisa and arranged an appointment to see me in Boston as soon as I could possibly get on a plane and be there.

Everything changed overnight. Larry showed up at the door to my room the next morning bringing me clothing and shoes, makeup, a hat, and a coat. My discharge paperwork was brought to my room while I got dressed. My personal belongings were returned, papers were signed, and I walked out the door holding Larry's hand past inmates catcalling to me. I didn't look back.

Once we were in the car, Larry explained to me that we would be driving straight to the airport and taking a flight to Boston as Dr. Mona Lisa had set up an appointment at Massachusetts General

Hospital for me. I called Dr. Mona Lisa and made her promise that I would not be admitted to another psychiatric ward. She reassured me by saying that Larry and I would be staying in a hotel across the street from Dr. Rosenbaum's office and she was catching a flight from Maine to meet up with us in Boston for the first appointment.

I felt weak, but I couldn't tell if it was from exhaustion or relief. The psychiatrist at UCLA had provided me with a medication to keep my anxiety in check as I made the flight from one coast to the other.

I opened the bag, feeling that I should take something before getting into the crowds at the airport. It was my ol' pal Klonopin, prescribed by the same psychiatrist who was supposedly completely familiar with my chart. How could I trust anyone with my care anymore? I kept the Klonopin out of Larry's sight and took one. I wasn't sure what would be my fate in the hands of yet another psychiatrist in Boston and I wanted the security of something that made me feel peaceful and calm. Forty minutes later, when the pilot came over the speakers to tell all the passengers to "sit back and relax and enjoy your six-hour-and-twenty-three-minute flight into Boston," I thought it was the best therapeutic advice I had been given in a month.

Chapter 16

Somewhere, Upon Some Bright New Dawn…

On the flight into Boston I paged through a newsmagazine featuring the overdose death of mega-talented actor Philip Seymour Hoffman. He reportedly had had a drug addiction problem in his early twenties and in an earlier interview was quoted as saying that he would take "anything I could get my hands on. I liked it all." He and his longtime girlfriend and mother to his three children separated at the end of 2013 and she had custody of the kids. Earlier in the year he had relapsed after decades of sobriety and admitted himself for rehab. He was there for ten days. I was curious to know if he had been given a benzodiazepine when he was discharged. Hoffman died of a heroin overdose. Some people made judgmental comments about his death: "How could he? He was so talented and successful?"

Six years earlier I might have been one of the people who asked those questions. Not anymore. I understood the destructive power that depression and anxiety can have and how dependence on a drug can set you free of your own thoughts, at least for a little while. There's the hook. The "little while" turns into a month, then a year, then one more year. You can no longer imagine feeling fine on a daily basis, or even remember what your life used to be. Once you can no longer hold the hope of feeling like things will get better, there is no motivation to stay away from drugs like Klonopin, even though it's supposed to be prescribed as a very short-term medication.

I peered out of the window as the plane banked over Boston Harbor. The water was choppy and dark gray, roughly slapping the edges of the concrete piers. Winter cold had stripped the trees bare and long late afternoon shadows from the buildings made the city below seem as tired and dispirited as I felt.

I held Larry's hand as the plane bounced down on the runway and the force of the brakes seemed to push me forward to yet another new course of treatment, another psychiatric opinion, another therapy method, another desperate grasp at finding a solution to my state of mental distress. I didn't really want to be there. It had been an emotional respite to be "nowhere," just thirty-five thousand feet in the sky, moving at five hundred miles per hour, as if I didn't belong on the earth.

Larry and I checked into the hotel and soon after Dr. Mona Lisa arrived in time to go with us to meet with Dr. Jerrold Rosenbaum. It had already been a long day and I was feeling anxious about having to talk to a new psychiatrist. I didn't want to appear too crazy and had a tremendous fear that he would recommend I be hospitalized again.

Dr. Mona Lisa knew how incredibly busy Dr. Rosenbaum is, but after he looked at my thick chart, his curiosity was piqued and he wanted to take me on as a patient.

Dr. Rosenbaum oversees a department of over seven hundred faculty members, including psychologists, psychiatrists, neuroscientists and well over a hundred trainees. He has written or edited twenty books and many scholarly articles with a special interest in people who suffer from previously treatment-resistant psychiatric problems. After Dr. Mona Lisa explained all of that to me, I felt very honored that he would consider seeing me as his patient. Because of his leadership role and caseload, Dr. Rosenbaum is unable to accept new patients.

I felt both comfortable and in very good hands as soon as I met this attractive man with a gentle, sincere voice and manner. I could see as he sat across from me that he wasn't going to treat me like a powerless child, but would expect me to participate in my own care. I felt something I hadn't known in a long time—hope. My shoulders relaxed as I sank back into my chair.

That night, in the hotel room, I was certain I would be able to sleep calmly since I was free of the noise of the psychiatric ward at UCLA, but that wasn't to be. I had a powerful anxiety attack that made me jump to my feet.

Our hotel room had a bathroom with two doors, one leading to a small sitting area and the other into the bedroom. There was also a door between the sitting area and the bedroom. I could walk a full circle, from the sitting area through the bedroom, through the bathroom, and back to the sitting area. As I paced this circle, my mind ran rampant, my heart beating wildly. I was consumed with worry about heading into yet another program or treatment. My body felt like such a dumping ground for too many medications that had not helped me. I could only guess at what Dr. Rosenbaum would try. Could I survive yet another round of trial-and-error? I didn't want to merely be tranquilized as a way out of pain, but I was losing hope that anything would help.

As it turned out, Dr. Rosenbaum's first suggestion was not for another medication. It was for me to stay in the Boston area for the next three weeks and start treatment rounds of electroconvulsive therapy there at Mass General. The words made me gasp. Having a convulsion because of electricity coursing through my brain seemed like such an extreme measure.

Dr. Rosenbaum assured me that it wasn't like the horrific treatments that actress Frances Farmer went through in the 1940s, or the ECT depicted in the film *One Flew Over the Cuckoo's Nest*. There had been decades of study and modernization of the technique since then and ECT treatment was now relatively low risk and shown to be successful for depression like mine that wasn't responding to regular medications. Still, my legs bounced up and down with nervousness and my palms broke out in sweat with the thought of having a seizure induced by electricity.

I could see that Dr. Rosenbaum was studying my every movement as I sat across from him in his office. He took the time to explain to me all of the long-range side effects of the huge amounts of benzos I had ingested in the past year and why continuing on them was not advisable. He also voiced his concern about my having been on so many antidepressants, none of which had helped me. Dr. Rosenbaum felt that my severe treatment-resistant depression was affecting my overall health and he was greatly concerned about my having suicidal ideations for over two years.

ECT has a strong and immediate effect on the neurotransmitters in the brain. It's the minute-long seizure that changes the neural networks, the biological abnormalities, which are associated with depression. The modified seizure would make changes in the brain centers that control moods, appetite, and sleep. Typically, patients need six or more treatments to see a noticeable improvement.

The main side effect of the treatments was a possible loss of short-term memory for a while; usually patients can't remember what happened in the time right before the treatment. The stack of release papers and informed consent forms that I had to sign prior to having an ECT treatment was intimidating, especially when I had to struggle just to keep our hotel room number in my memory. Wading through the "what could go wrong" pages on these forms was more than I could absorb. I signed everything, only reading some of it. In the darkness of depression, you give up caring what they do to you. You are willing to try anything to get out of the constant pain.

I was sent back to the hotel with instructions to have no food or liquids after midnight. I couldn't take any medication at all, but benzodiapenes especially were not permitted because of how they might interact with the general anesthesia. I had been counting on being able to take a Klonopin to help minimize my apprehension and anxiety about the first treatment early the next morning. All night long I paced the oval track from the bathroom to the sitting area to the bedroom, around and around.

The next morning, a nurse had me change into a hospital gown, took my blood pressure, checked my heart rate with a monitor, and inserted the IV needle. It was an assembly line atmosphere, with a patient before me, and another after me. I waited my turn, wary of how casual the technicians were. What if they make a mistake? What if I lose all my memory and become what I fear most, a woman who can't take care of herself?

Soon I was wheeled into a room of the outpatient psych unit of Mass General, where a doctor, nurse, and anesthesiologist were waiting. The nurse placed thick padded straps across my upper chest and on my legs above my knees, which secured my body to the bed as the doctor explained the procedure one more time and how quickly it goes. Two electrode pads were placed on my head, one on each temple. The doctor said about sixty seconds of electrical current would pass through the lobes of my brain, causing a controlled seizure.

He kindly rested his hand on my shoulder and looked in my eyes as he talked. The nurse put in a mouthguard to keep me from biting down hard on my teeth or my tongue during the seizure. Then the anesthesiologist added the "knockout" drugs to my IV. I was told to count backward from one hundred, but I don't remember doing that. I was out.

When I came to, it took a few minutes to understand where I was and what had taken place. A nurse was asking me my full name and if I knew what day of the week it was, to make sure that my memory was intact.

The first physical sensation I felt was that the bed below me was wet and I was uncomfortably damp from the waist down. It took me another minute to realize that I was lying in my own urine. I couldn't believe that had happened. No one had told me to make certain that my bladder was completely empty before changing into a hospital gown. I was humiliated to the core.

I was tired and spacey and only wanted to wash up, get dressed, and go back to the hotel. The muscles in my legs felt as shaky as if I had hiked a steep hill. My arms also shook, as if from muscle fatigue.

My short-term memory proved to be fine, so I was released for the day and told to come back in three days. This was to be my life for the next eighteen days: have a treatment, recover from it, and then return for another. I had short appointments with Dr. Rosenbaum so he could see how I was progressing. I didn't notice much change after the first three treatments. He told me that people with profoundly severe depression, like mine, might not feel the remission of symptoms for at least six to twelve treatments, maybe more.

After the fourth ECT treatment, Larry took me back to the hotel room to rest. I was starving. I hadn't had a bite to eat since an early dinner the night before. I ordered a stack of pancakes with a side of eggs from room service and looked forward to having a big breakfast.

We set up the room service table near the window to get the full effect of the little bit of Boston winter sunlight that had found its way to our side of the building. I buttered the pancakes and poured syrup over the top. When I took my first bite, I almost choked on the putrid taste. I had to spit it out on the plate. The pancake tasted the way raw sewage smells. I pushed it all away from me. I told Larry that someone in the room service kitchen had played a disgusting prank on me, somehow making the pancakes look normal while adding some type of rancid and nauseating ingredients that would make me violently ill. The room service manager apologized profusely, saying that he was astounded that something like that had happened, and said he would send up another breakfast right away.

The second serving of pancakes tasted as bad as the first batch.

Larry decided to try the pancakes himself. It was obvious that he didn't share my experience of the taste at all. He said they were delicious and ate the whole stack.

I tried a bite of the eggs and had to spit those out as well. A wave of panic set in.

What had happened to my sense of taste? I definitely couldn't eat anything on the plate. All I could do was hope that it was a temporary side effect of the ECT treatment and that it would go away. I had been warned about the risk of memory loss, but not about having my sense of taste go haywire.

The next morning Dr. Rosenbaum responded that in all of his years at the hospital he had never known a patient to have their taste buds altered through ECT treatments. Dr. Mona Lisa had never heard of it, either, but said she would look into it. We sent emails to all the doctors and scientists we could think of, who in turn forwarded them on to every professional they knew. No one had ever heard of taste buds being so adversely affected.

I did notice some subtle improvement in my state of mind. I wasn't sure if it was the ECT treatments, or having my freedom back after being locked up in UCLA's psychiatric ward. I started to look forward to bundling up and taking a walk with Larry around the Beacon Hill area. I found myself seeing and appreciating pleasant things: kids playing, dogs wagging their tails, and boats docked in the harbor. Most noticeably, I found that my suicidal thoughts had been pushed out of the daily lineup of thoughts I had to fight against. The ECT treatments did seem to increase my willingness to participate in life once again.

The major disappointment was being in a great food city like Boston and unable to eat anything that didn't taste putrid. I had to resort to drinking smoothies mixed with protein powder, because I could just swallow them and not have to taste them. Every morning I had a hopeful anticipation that my sense of taste would return, but each day brought repeated disappointment. I became frightened that this would now be my new "normal."

The gradual lifting of the fog around my depression was a relief by day, but the anxiety at night was still relentless. I would be able to doze off for an hour and then wake up suddenly with a crushing feeling of fear. It was nearly impossible for Larry to sleep with my constant pacing in a circle. I would feel trapped in the hotel room, but going outside on the frozen streets at 1 a.m. was not an option.

Following my sixth ECT treatment, Dr. Rosenbaum did an assessment of my progress. He recommended that I continue with an ECT treatment program through an outpatient psych unit connected to Vanderbilt University Medical Center so that I could go home. I gladly agreed to the plan. I wanted to sleep in my own bed, surround myself with my four dogs, and see my friends again, which was taken as a positive sign by everyone.

I was missing Ashley and hoping for the chance to reconnect with Wy. Elijah, my grandson, was sending me texts to hurry home. He wrote that he was missing my cooking him pork chops, mashed potatoes and gravy, and corn on the cob. Time used to pass quickly and joyfully when I was out on a tour, but the past three months had seemed more like three decades.

Before I left Boston, we had a meeting with Dr. Rosenbaum about my panic at night and sleep issues. Sleep is paramount to helping the brain deal with depression. Without it, the amygdala, the area of the brain that controls the "fight or flight" survival instinct, goes into overdrive. You use less of the prefrontal cortex, which helps you apply reason and logic to whatever you're experiencing and keeps you calm.

Dr. Rosenbaum went over a list of suggestions that he calls "sleep hygiene," which he felt would lead to better rest for me:

1. Go to bed at the same time every night.
2. Rise at the same time every morning, even if you didn't sleep well during the night.
3. Choose some type of regular exercise and stick with it. Daily regular exercise improves the quality of sleep.
4. Keep the temperature in the bedroom cool, if possible.
5. Don't watch TV, especially late night news, or look at a computer screen in bed. The light stimulates activity in your mind.
6. Turn out all the lights and keep the bedroom quiet to facilitate good sleep.

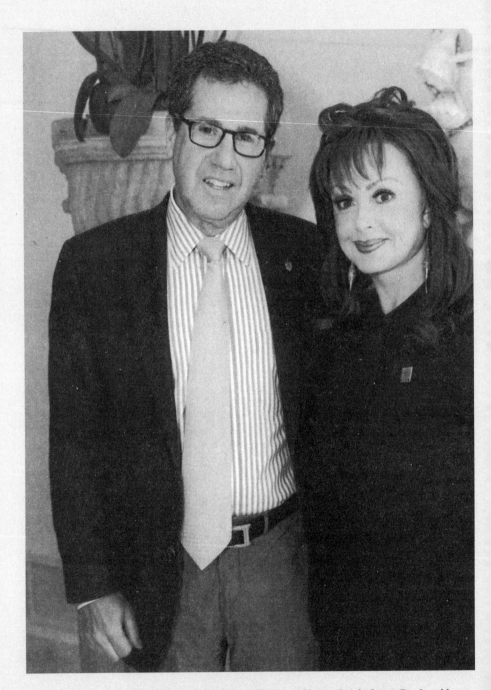

The man who I credit with the fact that I'm still alive and have a bright future, Dr. Jerrold Rosenbaum, chief of psychiatry at Massachusetts General Hospital in Boston.

7. Don't review problems in your head. Use a relaxation exercise or think about a recent pleasant experience.
8. Try a warm bath and listen to calming music before bed.
9. No napping during the day. (This one was problematic for me since I rarely slept during the night. Along with the list, he gave me a prescription for a light sleeping pill.)

"Will these nighttime panic attacks ever end?" I asked Dr. Rosenbaum. "They make me feel like I'm suffering a psychotic break."

Dr. Rosenbaum nodded in sympathy. "It's not a realistic fear. You're generating your own fear of fear. You will learn to float through it, and you'll start sleeping. Do deep breathing. Eventually you'll fall asleep. Most importantly, stay in the bed, so you can let your mind realize that the panic won't harm you. You won't die. You'll get through this."

He made it sound so simple. And it used to be. I would get in bed, read a few pages of a book, and I'd be out for seven or eight hours. Now my deep sadness and traumatic past were erupting like Old Faithful every single night.

As Larry and I went through the security at Logan International Airport, a woman on the other side of the line caught my eye. She reminded me of one of my mother's very few friends, Martha Compton. Her daughter, Hattie Lou, had been my brother Brian's age and had died of the exact same type of lymphoma six months before he did.

A few years later, Mother met Martha Compton when she started working at the town's small gift shop, the Aladdin, following her divorce from Daddy. They formed a special bond, both being mothers who had lost a teenage child to the same kind of cancer. Martha was certain that Brian and Hattie Lou had died from the effects of toxins in the air and water from the chemical plants in Ashland.

After Mother became friends with Martha, she shared these words with me, only once, when I was on a visit home to Ashland. "Naomi, always be nice to everyone, because you never know what they are going through personally." I knew she was talking about herself and her misery after my father moved out, but those words came back to me at Logan as I watched this woman who looked so much like Martha Compton walk away while other travelers started to approach me for autographs and photos.

As I smiled and posed for pictures with people who asked on the way to our gate, I thought about my mother's advice in terms of what I was going through and what others expected me to be. I'm certain each of these dear fans would find it hard to believe that I had just received six electroconvulsive treatments for severe depression, or that I had been hospitalized three times in psychiatric wards. Could they imagine the number of times I had pondered if today would be the day I jumped from a bridge? Would they ever guess that I was grasping for a miracle to save my own life? No, they wouldn't. I tried hard not to show any of it. I wanted their experience of me to be positive. I wanted to be Superstar Naomi Judd again and not this frightened woman, cowering under the attack of so much unresolved trauma in my life.

As Larry and I settled into our seats, rays of sun spilled through the window and onto my lap. I wanted to lie down and sleep in this warmth and forget about everything I had gone through. It's odd what the mind chooses to retain, years and years later, even if it has only experienced it once. From a long-ago memory file, I remembered the inscription on the sympathy card Martha Compton sent to Mother on the day after Brian died, but years before she and my mother met.

"Somewhere, upon some bright new dawn, the beautiful soul of him is bursting with eager joy."

Would there be a "bright new dawn" in my life? Could I feel an "eager joy" again? Did I dare to hope the ECT treatments would work to unscramble my worn and battered brain?

Chapter 17

Radical Acceptance

I am putting my brain in their hands! The thought of it made me anxious every single time I had electroconvulsive therapy at the outpatient psych unit at Vanderbilt hospital in Nashville. The records show that things go wrong in hospitals all the time. What if I lose my memory?

Every three days, Larry would wake me up at 7 a.m. and drive me into Nashville for another treatment. We always went first thing in the morning before I had any breakfast or even a cup of coffee, which I really didn't miss since none of it tasted good to me.

I would see the same group of psych patients, awaiting their own ECT treatments, when I arrived for my appointments. The group ranged in age from the late seventies to a teenage girl. I knew they each had a story of what brought them to this point, the same way I did. But depression is a solo disease. As we all waited our turn for treatment, a sad silence hung over the room.

I had the same IV anesthesiologist, who delivered the knock-out drug, at each appointment. He would rest his hand gently on my shoulder and solemnly assure me, "We're going to take really good care of you. Don't worry."

I would say to him, "Now, make sure you tell me before you put me to sleep. I want to be in control of this one thing." I would try to count and see how far I got before the powerful drug would put me under. There was a relief in those few seconds before becoming unconscious. My body had no choice but to relax, and for that brief pause in time I was free of my depression and anxiety.

Later, as we were driving back to our farm, I thought about Michael Jackson's death and how he reportedly begged his doctor to administer propofol, a surgical anesthetic, so he could be unconscious for a while. As extreme as that request seemed to most people, in my current state of mind I could comprehend why he wanted the medication. Trying to prepare for his massive final world tour must have been a terrible pressure. Tickets had sold out around the world and expectations were sky-high. Could the fifty-year-old Michael still wow an audience like the twenty-five-year-old Michael? Every decision was his to make. As his family described it, he was having an impossible time turning off his anxious mind and sleeping.

More performers than you would suspect suffer debilitating effects from anxiety, stage fright, insomnia, or depression. Long before I had my own issues, ironically, I would sometimes be called upon to console other artists who were being held back by fears.

My friend the singer-songwriter Carly Simon has been public about her panic attacks since the mid-1980s. When she first started to tour again, she would call me from backstage right before her concert. Because of my nursing career and my own personal suffering, I had developed ways of helping others through anxiety. When you get nervous, your shoulders rise up and your stomach caves in, which is the worst thing for a singer who needs all of her breath support. I would always call it "earrings" when Wy and I were backstage before a show. It was a signal that our shoulders were creeping up by our ears and not relaxed.

The advice I would give Carly was to take off her shoes, which kind of fit with her act anyway, and spread her toes wide. "Remember that you are connected with the great Mother Earth, Carly. Then rock your hips around to get more flexible and feel your energy flowing up and down. When you go onstage, make eye contact with your favorite band member, and go back to stand by him if you feel anxiety coming on. Let him know beforehand, so he can make eye contact."

Carly told me that she never wanted to be a performer, only a songwriter. It seems clear that our bodies react negatively to thoughts and experiences that are outside of our true wants and desires. Her desire was to stay off the stage, but she was under pressure from her record labels to do live shows. In contrast, my desire was to stay onstage, and my whole biological being seemed to be in turmoil because I had no alternative plan for when my career came to an abrupt end.

After the next six ECT treatments, I didn't notice any improvement in my depression, although I did think much less about putting a gun to my head or jumping off the bridge. Dr. Rosenbaum advised that I complete the course of ECT treatments, twelve more, as my depression had proven to be severely treatment resistant. For the next two months my life revolved around going to the ECT clinic once every three days and then needing a full day of recovery the day after, when I felt "zapped" of my energy. The following day I would feel better, but then would have to return for another treatment the next morning and repeat the three-day cycle. Larry continued to stay by my side, driving me back and forth for treatments. My heart went out to any of the other patients who lived alone or had to figure out how to manage without such support.

After one of my ECT treatments at Vanderbilt, the chair of the department of psychiatry came to check on me. I had been having a rough morning, and was in need of a strong dose of encouragement. When I asked this ultimate expert, "Am I going to make it?" He answered coldly, without pause, "I don't think so." That was it. I was flattened by a cruel and crushing proclamation of defeat. Following that day, I no longer believed in the ability of the ECT therapy to help heal my mind and I never went back.

*   *   *

Though the ECT treatments didn't affect my short-term memory, which is a side effect for some people, it did make my mind feel much more foggy and unfocused. This concerned me greatly because I still had a string of scheduled speeches on my calendar that I had committed to more than a year earlier. As tough as the speaking engagements had been for me prior to the ECT treatments, it was now even more frightening. I couldn't keep track of where I was in the delivery. In many ways, I was feeling like a novice in unfamiliar territory, though I've been a keynote speaker for years. Before my depression treatments, I was able to talk for forty-five minutes with only a brief outline on one piece of paper. Now it became a laborious process for me. My assistant would have to organize and set up PowerPoint slides so that I could remember the direction the speech needed to go. Without them, I might find myself meandering off topic. For many of the groups in the health care profession, my keynote speech served as part of their mandatory continuing education units. This piled on the pressure since I had been brought in to expand the foundation of knowledge for the attending professionals and keep them up-to-date on new developments. Somehow I pulled it off.

My taste buds were still missing in action three months after that fourth ECT treatment. I could no longer enjoy any food at all. One evening, Larry and I went to a popular Mexican restaurant in town. I thought that perhaps the more spicy flavors would override the bad taste, but it made it worse. The food tasted like chemicals to me. I couldn't take more than two bites. The salsa had looked delicious, but it tasted as though it was laced with Windex, and the chip tasted like burnt plastic.

I wanted to leave as soon as possible. I became even more wary of eating anything in public after this unsuccessful outing. I know most of the restaurant owners and chefs in our small town and didn't want them to feel it was their fault that I couldn't eat what I had ordered. They'd often come over to our table to ask what was wrong with my barely touched plate of food.

I found myself left with only a very few choices for nutrition. I could manage to swallow a tablespoon of peanut butter for protein, and drink smoothies for fruits and veggies, and that was my limit. Other foods would make me feel like gagging. I started to lose weight rapidly, about two pounds each week. Not a diet I would recommend to anyone! Taste buds are something we all take for granted and having them misfire, making everything taste horrible, added to my anxious feelings that I would never have a normal life again.

About a month after the ECT treatments ended, I could tell that I was slowly falling back into thoughts of suicide. After three major hospitalizations, an outpatient program, a cavalcade of prescription medicines, one right after another, and twenty-four ECT treatments, I didn't see that I had gained much ground at all. In fact, I seemed to be adding more unnerving symptoms. Besides my distorted sense of taste making it impossible to eat, I was having a visible symptom that made me never want to leave the safety of my kitchen couch. My hair began shedding by the handful. Every time I brushed my hair, more fell out.

I had always had thick, wavy, auburn hair, which was the physical feature I liked most about myself. Losing most of my once-glorious head of hair increased my feelings of hopelessness. The only place I could be without wearing a hat or a full wig was my own house. When I visited my doctor and had to remove my hat, the people in the office questioned what type of cancer treatment I was undergoing.

My fervent hopes of patching up my relationship with Wynonna seemed more faint than ever. Since I still didn't want her to see me in my current condition, I didn't reach out to her, either. One of the brightest lights in my relentless sorrow was my grandson, Elijah, who would come over at night with a stack of funny videos or movies that we would watch together. He could tell that I was in a hole once again. His steady and caring nature gave me reason to hang in there day by day, though I could no longer imagine any future that would hold hope. Even the spring and summer days with their longer hours of daylight didn't help much to boost my increasing sense of taking a one-way street to an early end.

Dr. Rosenbaum checked in with me by phone at least twice a week. After listening to my voice, he strongly urged me to travel back to Boston for an appointment. He wanted to see me, in person, to note how I appear physically. He told me that direct observation reassures him more than just hearing my voice on the phone, so observing me was paramount to his decision making.

During electroconvulsive therapy, the protocol is for the patient to abstain from taking certain types of psychiatric-based medications. It was now clear that the ECT had not provided consistent improvement for me. Dr. Rosenbaum decided to take a totally different approach with my medications, since no antidepressants had previously worked. He started me on high daily dosages of Parnate, an MAOI (monoamine oxidase inhibitor). He explained that it's an old-school second-line treatment that works best for people with major depressive disorders combined with extreme anxiety. The MAOIs have been around since the mid-1950s and are not often used for depression anymore because of the dangers of fatal interactions with foods or other medications. I was sternly warned that I couldn't eat or drink anything containing high levels of tyramine, which is derived from the amino acid tyrosine. I was given an entire list of foods that the drug could react with and possibly kill me. This includes anything fermented or aged: wine, cheese, smoked meats, soy products, and others. Sadly, included on this list was chocolate.

He also decided to prescribe lithium, an element found in traces in granite, other types of rock, seawater, and mineral hot springs. Lithium carbonate is the form used for psychiatric drugs. It is mainly indicated as a mood stabilizer for mood swings but is thought by some to potentiate or add to the efficacy of antidepressants. It has many properties that affect brain activity and neuronal signaling but why it can work is still mainly unknown. Like Parnate, it comes with certain dietary cautions like too much or too little salt and excessive caffeine intake. The Lithium levels also have to be monitored through having blood tests, as too high of levels are toxic to our biology.

About seven days after beginning both prescriptions, I could feel a slight change, a peek at a new dawn on the horizon. It wasn't a dramatic difference. It was more like a spark of stability that was within my sight. For the first time in two and a half years, I could sense the possibility of ascending from, instead of descending deeper into, a dark and lifeless hole. I was also prescribed many other medications.

While I was in Boston, Dr. Rosenbaum was very direct with me about facing and accepting where I was in my life. Without an ounce of cruelty in his voice, he asked very direct questions about my unwillingness to face some of the new realities of life as time had passed, since I had done the work to face my long suppressed traumas. He wanted to bring me into the present.

"How did you imagine life would be as you got older? Did you think about a new normal with respect to beauty and fame as you aged? Did you not consider that Wynonna would want to sing solo going forward? Do you understand that it is too late to be a failure because you have already acquired such a lifetime of success? Can you hold in your thoughts the awareness of all you have done, where you have been, and the joys still ahead? You have insatiable curiosity. Aren't you getting tired of only grieving what is passed?"

It was like having a bucket of cold water dumped over my head, shocking me out of my evaporating daydream. I was angry as hell because he struck a nerve of truth. He was right. I was clinging, desperately, to a past that I wanted to continue into the present. It wasn't going to be and I had no other choice than to face it. After many tests, observations, interviews, and meetings with Larry, Dr. Rosenbaum, and Dr. Mona Lisa, I was diagnosed with severe treatment-resistant depression. Meaning they had tried everything they could think of and nothing was working.

Dr. Rosenbaum firmly suggested that in conjunction with the prescription medicines, I start working with a therapist trained in dialectical behavior therapy. He assured me that it didn't need to be in a hospital setting and that there were qualified people in the Nashville area and across the United States.

I had participated in cognitive behavior therapy while doing outpatient therapy at PCS in Arizona. It's a method of treatment that focuses on altering your current thought process for the better and changing behaviors that are causing you to suffer emotionally. I wasn't aware of dialectical behavior therapy.

The word *dialectical* refers to the way the mind understands a concept by recognizing its polar opposite. As a simple example, we wouldn't understand the concept of daylight if we didn't experience the darkness of nighttime.

Psychologist Marsha Linehan developed dialectical behavior therapy in response to people who weren't being helped by cognitive behavioral therapy. It's a tried-and-true evidence-based therapy, particularly created for people with suicidal ideation, people who chronically have thoughts of ending their emotional anguish with death.

DBT starts with actively accepting and validating the patient no matter what the current state of mind is, even if the patient is suicidal. First the therapist works on acceptance and then begins to incorporate change, especially for clients with low distress tolerance. Instead of teaching clients how to change, the goal for dialectical behavior therapy is to help clients learn to "radically accept" where they are and learn to tolerate stress and distress. The therapist works as an ally, keeping the patient participating in her own therapy by learning problem-solving skills, and then validating the client's efforts.

The therapy is a comprehensive treatment that has worked for many emotional problems and mental health issues. It has proven highly successful for people with traumatic childhoods like mine. One of the concepts of DBT that isn't part of most therapies is traumatic invalidation.

Traumatic invalidation happens when you feel invalidated or ignored for the person you are, what you do, and what you think, by people who matter greatly to you. When someone important to you invalidates you, parents specifically, you can still be traumatized by shame, anger, and deep hurt decades later and it continues to influence how you react to current life experiences.

This was my entire childhood, living in an extended family, both maternal and paternal, of people with no relationship skills or ability to express their true feelings in a healthy way. And it was also my current life.

I could no longer feel validated as a performer. Wynonna was no longer into the Judds as her career direction. She was busy creating Wynonna and the Big Noise. Many of the fans moved over to follow her new direction. I believed I was thought of only as a nostalgic memory and it hurt badly. Also, Wy and I were out of tune with each other personally, and I missed her desperately.

I went back to the farm, knowing that I would have to figure out how to find peace in the present and create a new future; otherwise I would never heal my depression and anxiety. I saw a couple of DBT therapists both privately and in a group setting, but didn't feel comfortable in either situation. In a group setting, I fell into the trap of wanting to "help" others too much, because it's my nature. This was detrimental for my therapeutic purpose, as I needed to deal with my own issues and not distract myself with the problems of others. I began to get discouraged, my self-esteem dipped lower, and I questioned if I would ever find the right therapist.

Dr. Rosenbaum encouraged me to keep searching, trying out different therapists. He stressed that a therapist you can trust is crucial to the process. If you're working with someone who makes you feel uneasy, you will find yourself holding back. The right balance is to find a therapist who makes you feel safe, but who will also challenge you to move beyond the thoughts that are keeping you stuck in your depression or anxiety.

After a few months of mismatches, I found my wonderful DBT therapist, Diana Partington. She recognized right away that I was in a vulnerable and defeated state of mind, so we began our session there. She is a great combination of gentle, caring warmth and dedicated and persuasive coach, who absolutely expects me to rise to my potential.

The creator of DBT, Marsha Linehan, published a workbook with valuable information and actual homework to do between sessions with your therapist. It's a toolkit of skills to use to both self-validate and in reaction to other people and emotional circumstances. Instead of digging deep into the unconscious and analyzing how you came to be where you are, DBT helps you get through your present day and the near future, reducing your vulnerability to your emotions, by teaching skills to increase certain behaviors, some of which are listed in the workbook as "ABC PLEASE."

A: ACCUMULATE POSITIVE EMOTIONS: I began to incorporate such emotion into my life by choosing to do things that are pleasant and possible today. Also, Diana encouraged me to make changes so that more positive events would happen in my future.

B: BUILD MASTERY: Find something that you feel strongly or passionate about. Choose something that makes you feel effective and competent. The purpose of this is to move you away from a feeling of hopelessness.

C: COPE AHEAD OF TIME WITH EMOTIONAL SITUATIONS: Have a plan in mind if you are heading into a situation that makes you emotional. This skill helps you feel less helpless.

PLEASE: TAKE CARE OF YOUR MIND BY TAKING

CARE OF YOUR BODY. Balance nutritious eating, plenty of sleep, and daily exercise with having any physical illnesses treated.

Diana met with me weekly, as I slowly began to apply the methods of emotional regulation suggested by DBT. I still had long weeks of immobility, as new side effects of taking Parnate, lithium, and the other medications began to appear. Though Parnate was the first medication that proved to have an effect on my depression, it was not without a price. The Parnate continued to cause my hair loss. By the end of summer, I was left with a ponytail about as thick as you might see on a fourteen-month-old baby, and Parnate made my cheeks puffy. In addition, the lithium gave my hands a tremor that was worse in the morning and a bit better later in the day. If I had to meet with anyone, I would hide my hands under the table or behind me.

I could no longer write with a pen in a legible way. My penmanship looked wavy and wobbled off in random directions, the result of my hand shaking uncontrollably. Beginning in grade school, people had always complimented me on my nice handwriting. Like my hair, it was always a source of pride and one of my attributes I appreciated the most. (A Nashville radio DJ once told Wynonna, "I want to show you something." From his desk drawer he pulled out a handwritten thank-you note I had sent to him early in our career, after he took a chance and played our newly released first song on his station. He told Wy that he had held on to it all these years because he rarely gets thank-you notes from artists and my handwriting was beautiful.)

Losing both my handwriting ability and my hair made me feel that God Himself was testing me like Job. What else would vanish from my life? My career had evaporated. Sleeping for more than a couple of hours a night was next to impossible. My oldest daughter was out of touch with me. Mother appeared to be oblivious to anything I was going through. I had lost millions of dollars to a swindler business partner. And now my hair and my ability even to sign my name were vanishing, leaving me to feel I was dispossessed of many things that had defined me for most of my life.

As a dialectical behavior therapist Diane didn't deny my feelings. She wanted to know "why I wanted to end it." I answered, "I want God to end this pain." She explained to me that when things are really, really bad, it's easy to romanticize suicide as an escape hatch. You begin to think that everything will be better once it's all over. Then she asked me, bluntly, "So, what do you think happens after you die? Is it going to be better? The Bible and most religions don't look favorably upon suicide. Do you have any guarantees that it's going to be better?" I didn't have an answer for her.

Diana pulled her chair closer and promised, "I can give you a guarantee of something. I can guarantee, one hundred percent, that there are going to be better days than this one. You know it's true because you've had them. And you've had bad days like this one and survived to live a better day."

I nodded in agreement, but I still had nothing to say.

"If you kill yourself," Diana pressed on, "there's no guarantee. But if you stay here and stick with it and climb out of this, I can help you."

Linehan uses the metaphor of climbing out of hell on a steel ladder. It burns. It hurts as you go up. "This is your climb out of hell, Naomi," Diana said. "It will get easier as you go higher. But you will never know that if you kill yourself."

I wanted so badly to believe Diana's guarantee. Severe depression had made me irrational. There was no feeling of vitality with depression and the pain creates thoughts of darkness that feel abso-lutely real. I needed this connectivity with Diana. At a time when I couldn't trust my own irrational thoughts, I found I could trust hers. It helped me get through each week until we met again.

When I first started seeing Diana as a therapist, I would have some appointments at my house and some in her office. One morn-ing, I realized I had forgot an appointment that was scheduled that day in her office. Hurriedly I taped a note to the door for Larry, who had gone to play golf.

I headed out the door, turning off my cell phone for the hourlong appointment. After our session, I forgot to turn my cell phone back on. About a mile from our farm, I saw Larry driving toward me. His face was completely pale and his eyes looked frantic. Something had to be horribly wrong and it made me panic, too. Larry made a sharp U-turn and followed me to our driveway. As I got out of the car I saw that Larry looked as if he could drop to his knees on the driveway. I now knew his panic had been about me.

"Where have you been? I've been calling and calling you," Larry demanded

I explained that I was running late and had taped a note to the door. When I turned on my cell phone back on, there were seven messages from Larry. The final one warned that if he didn't hear back from me in five minutes, he was going to contact the sheriff's office.

As it turns out, ninety minutes earlier, Larry had not found my note when he arrived home. After searching the house and noticing that my car was gone, he tried my cell phone. When it went directly to my voice mail, Larry's mind jumped to the worst conclusion. He had driven at top speed to the Natchez Trace Parkway Bridge, afraid that today was the day I had chosen to leap to my death.

I don't think I'll ever forget the look on my husband's face at the thought of me making that choice. There was no happy ending or relief with suicide. I could easily end my own life, but it didn't mean that misery would die with me. It would be like the ash from the giant furnaces at the production plants in my hometown of Ashland. My misery would settle like a dark layer of grief over everyone I left behind.

Actor and comedian Robin Williams had committed suicide earlier in the fall and that evening I thought about one of my interactions with him backstage a number of years earlier. We were both performing for the same charity event.

Whenever I participated in a variety or late-night show, I always arrived with my hair and makeup already done and dressed in the outfit I was going to wear onstage. I liked to have the time to leave my dressing room door open so I could chat with the other performers.

I could hear Robin's voice in the hallway as he careened from dressing room to dressing room, and the trail of loud laughter that followed him to my door. He came in, twirling my makeup chair on its stand, making faces into the mirror, and running through a dozen character voices, and then pulling a pair of pantyhose over his head trying to make me laugh. But it wasn't a real interaction with me. It was a manic and irrepressible display. It soon made me feel very nervous in its bombardment of energy practically bouncing off the walls. After about five minutes I finally took Robin's forearm and cajoled, "Hey, guy, you've got to split because you're winding me up too much. I've got to sing and I can't when I feel all hyper." With that he bounded out of my dressing room and into the one next door.

I had remembered that a sound tech who had worked on the crew of *Mrs. Doubtfire* had mentioned how manic Robin was the entire time they were filming. He exhausted his cast-mates and crew, and everyone wanted to tell Robin to "calm down."

In retrospect, I remembered noticing how sad Robin's eyes were, even though he was constantly "on" and bigger than life. I certainly didn't know Robin well enough to make any assumptions about his inner life. After having such a long, ongoing depression myself, I wondered if, like me, he had traumatic emotional memories that were demanding his attention. Were his brilliant, quick-witted mind and luminous personality that never took a break in public all a coping mechanism to keep the trauma submerged? Was that an impossible feat once his life slowed down following his heart surgery, and as he secretly suffered with diffuse Lewy body dementia, which had gone undiagnosed for far too long?

I appreciated reading this quote from actress and writer Carrie Fisher about Robin: "He was driven by that frantic eagerness that you don't just want someone to like you, you want to explode on their night sky like a miracle. And he did."

I thought about how many creative artists commit suicide, either knowingly or by overdose or fatal mixture of drugs, without considering the consequences. Creative people need to have a way to express their vision, to have a purpose and a goal. Depression can cause you to believe that you have no artistic vision or future, which can make a creative person feel hopelessly dead inside.

When Dr. Mona Lisa called to check in on me over the weekend, I told her, "I don't care how many years I have left in my life. I only want those years to have purpose, meaning, and joy."

As Diana, my therapist, would tell me during every session, I needed to radically accept where my life was right now and slowly build it back into a life worth living. As she explained it: Radical acceptance is to know that painful things are still going to happen, but how we respond makes a difference. We don't have to condone our current reality, but we have to accept it for what it is instead of staying stuck, wishing it were different. Pain will happen, but suffering is optional. You can change your future reality, but you first have to accept the present reality.

It was time to really work the ABC, PLEASE plan. DBT would become a big part of my salvation.

Chapter 18
What Michelangelo Knew

couldn't be alone. Being alone terrified me and created panic. If Larry couldn't be with me, then someone had to come over and "babysit" me. This wasn't how I wanted to be. It was humiliating. But then, being alone was far worse for me than the humiliation.

The prolific writer Virginia Woolf knew about being alone. She wrote of "always some terror; so afraid one is of loneliness; of seeing to the bottom of the vessel." As long as someone was with me, I didn't have to examine the bottom of the vessel. Woolf saw the bottom and she drowned herself. I knew I had to prevent the opportunity for the disease in my brain to convince me of the logic of a similar fate. If I spent time alone, I would find myself ruminating constantly. I decided to accept that, until my oppressive depression and anxiety abated somewhat, I wouldn't be critical of myself for needing not to be alone. One of my lifelong emotional traumas has always been abandonment by Mother, Daddy, my relatives, my siblings, and my first husband.

One of the first things Diana advised me to do was make concrete plans for activities that helped me boost the number of positive emotions in my life. I had to begin to outweigh the overwhelming traumatic memories with good new memories. The traumatic memories couldn't be replaced, but they shouldn't have the ability to run and ruin my present-day life anymore. I had to work toward regulating the distressing emotions by replacing them with positive new actions. To break an old bad habit you must replace it with a better new one.

To address my feelings of loneliness, I decided to return to a tradition that I have always treasured, family dinners. I set a firm date on my calendar on every available Thursday to cook a big meal and have family and close friends over to eat.

If Ashley was in town, she came over with any guest she wanted to bring. One night she showed up with four of her girlfriends. My grandson, Elijah, and his longtime girlfriend, Haley, are mainstays. Often our dear friends Roy and Helen came. Tanner and Beatte, the brother and sister, who are the adult children of Wy's road manager, Tami, loved to be invited. They call Larry and me Papaw and Mamaw.

I would shop early in the morning and then spend almost the whole day cooking. When my family and friends were gathered around my dining table, I was able to forget my depression for an hour or two, even though I couldn't eat my own food because of my errant taste buds. I would still sit at the table with my smoothie.

My one firm rule for our Thursday family dinners was no cell phones at the table. Everyone seemed happy to comply. Actually "being" with each other, in person, with no technical distractions, was critical to my positive emotions about the evening. Social media might be a great way to catch up on one another's news, but I believe it has increased our feelings of separation drastically. Sitting behind a computer or staring down at a smartphone screen is not human interaction.

According to a study from Microsoft in the spring of 2015, our human attention span is now only eight seconds long! A goldfish has a longer attention span. How can we feel that we are seen or heard when we know that in eight seconds the other person's mind will wander? We are social beings. Interacting in person and not through a gadget changes our emotions and the nerve cells in our brains for the better.

At our Thursday dinners, Larry would ask a blessing over our food and then we all spent an hour or two talking about everything going on in our lives and in the world. Or we asked each other questions like "What is your biggest regret?" They produced revealing and insightful answers. Elijah and Ashley were surprised to learn that my biggest regret was that I didn't go to Iraq following 9/11 to work as a nurse.

It was always eye-opening to hear the perspective of the young people at the table about the current news headlines. And I like to think that Larry and I could give them perspective by relating some of our real-life experiences. Usually, only a matter of minutes would pass before someone said something hilarious and we all doubled over with gales of belly laughs.

At the end of the evening, my guests would take turns choosing what the menu would be for the next Thursday dinner. Once someone was invited to family dinner, they usually cleared their calendars to be a part of these regular Thursday evenings. The feeling of family, togetherness, and interaction with those I love helped me to remember that depression forces a person to look at life through a negative filter that isn't true reality.

Now, you may be thinking, Right. I wish I could have a family dinner without some type of drama or upset. Believe me, I understand. Nothing can bring me down quite as low as when there are family arguments. It makes me feel like there's no hope if my closest relationships aren't working. If your family has big personalities, like mine, it can be a challenge to keep the peace.

Years ago, early in my marriage to Larry, I came up with some simple family interaction rules called "Judd Family Powwow Rules." Larry, Wynonna, and Ashley also contributed. Then I had them printed up and laminated the page so that they can survive in the family kitchen without getting butter or mustard all over them. I can rinse the page off at the end of every meal. They worked for my family to make our time together better. Perhaps they will be beneficial for you, too.

The Judd Family Powwow Rules

1. No interrupting.
2. No shouting.
3. Each of us must realize we have our own realities.
4. Everyone gets as much time as they need to express themselves completely.
5. Everyone should be prepared with our thoughts and solutions, so time isn't wasted.
6. Stop and think before you speak so that you talk to the person as if he or she were a friend instead of a relative.
7. Everyone needs to remember that these are just issues. Our commitment to communicating is the bottom line to making sure the family endures.

And finally, conflict can't survive without your participation. Confrontation gets easier when you give up your need to be right. No matter how you slice it, there are always two sides.

One thing that contributed to my depression over time was the reality that I had only a very small family that I could count on as people who love me unconditionally, as I love them. This may be true for you, too. Or perhaps you have no actual blood relatives to count on as family.

My daughter Ashley came up with a great remedy for the longing for a large, close family. Every Sunday afternoon that she is in town Ashley hosts a picnic or get-together on her property. She invites the people she calls her "family of choice." Most of these people are people from our small village area who may not be geographically near any of their own relatives. The variety in the group keeps it lively: both couples and singles, artists, health care practitioners, humanitarian workers, soccer moms, yoga instructors, business owners, and intellectuals of all different ages, along with the young children of people in the group. Everyone brings a dish to share and we get involved in each other's lives, catching up on personal news in the same way family does.

Larry and I go if we are in town whenever possible. I get caught up in the enthusiasm of the little children and end up playing with them. I've been known to have a ring of dirt around my neck by the end of the picnic from my willingness to throw myself into any game. We play softball, dodgeball, badminton, and other games. We wade in the pond and collect moss for Ashley's garden.

There are always some interesting discussions to join in with the adults, a book recommendation, or even sharing something as helpful as how to get pen marks out of a white blouse.

Our "family of choice" relationships have extended beyond the Sunday picnic. We support each other in the ways a family would. We go to their kids' baseball games, celebrate birthdays, dive in to help when it's needed, and congratulate each other's successes. Larry and I attend the children's school events. We take them for pizza and ice cream afterward. We might meet a few other adults at a café or go to a movie together. In the past, we've all gone to the beach as a group and rented cabins on the shore.

This past winter we had a great snowfall over the weekend in the Nashville area. The valley on our property has a big sloping hill, perfect for sledding. The families were invited over and Larry got out our four-wheeler to bring the kids from the bottom of the hill back up to the top for another thrilling sled ride down. Their excitement and joy was like a happy virus that spread through my system, lifting my mood for the whole day. This chosen family has shown me how unconditional love can make a person feel accepted, safe, and useful.

I found I had become so isolated that I forgot that social interaction is the best way to be reminded that life is still going on in interesting ways. At first I had to push myself a bit to join back in socially, because it seemed as if my depression had zapped any ounce of energy I had. Some Sundays I couldn't imagine how I would figure out a dish to prepare and bring, because I felt so exhausted from depression or being up at night with a panic attack. However, the simple act of getting dressed, putting on a bit of makeup, and leaving the house would inevitably put me in a different frame of mind. Once I got going, I would forget that only one hour before I had been convinced I should stay home.

Depression also does a deceptive number on a person's self-esteem. I would often feel like I had nothing of interest to contribute to a group situation, or even a one-on-one with a friend. My mind would feel dull and scattered and I couldn't imagine engaging in a conversation that would matter to anyone. I found that my fears had no basis in reality. Most people are happy to have you listen. Listening will put new and different thoughts in your mind, and that alone will feel like a relief. You only have to ask a few questions and they will feel pleased that you are interested. Most people are paying attention to their own lives and are not sitting in judgment of you. Usually the best you can do is absolutely fine with them.

Besides doing one-to-one therapy with Diana, I found another outlet to talk about my feelings without the pressure of having to be careful about what I expressed. I began to attend Al-Anon meetings when I could. Al-Anon is a mutual support group for people who are or have been affected by someone who is an alcoholic. It is a twelve-step program and every meeting is confidential and anonymous. One of the main goals for people who attend Al-Anon meetings is to find ways to stop being codependent in a relationship with an alcoholic.

Though it was never spoken about or even labeled in my childhood home, Daddy was an extreme binge drinker on the weekends. He would never bring alcohol home, but would stay at his gas station after it closed for the day, and have a buddy or two come by and they would drink until dawn, by which point they were of course completely inebriated. I had no idea of this the entire time I lived at home, choosing instead in my adoration of Daddy to think that he was working extra-long hours on the weekends. He never went to church with us on Sunday. I would come downstairs, ready for breakfast and to go to Sunday school. Daddy would be sitting at the table, usually without a shirt on, his head propped in his hands and drinking a Pepsi. His eyes would be bloodshot and for some reason, most likely denial, I'd never notice that he could barely keep his head up because he was drunk. I remembered thinking, Poor Daddy. He works so hard. Mother would move noiselessly around the kitchen and then hustle us as quickly as possible out the door and off to church.

It was well into my adult life when I realized that I had grown up with an alcoholic father, which explained so much of his sullen moods, unwillingness to communicate, and separation from the family. What I understood is that I had picked up on Mother's cues to not press any buttons that might cause drama in the house. I learned my lessons well from her. I've had chronic codependency issues in my own relationships, which arose from my fear of being alone. My codependency has been the topic of many therapeutic hours for me. I could see how it contributed fully to my depression and anxiety once my performing career had lurched to a standstill.

There's a "home group" of about twenty-five people who gather for meetings, often in local churches. We make up a wide range of personalities and social status. One man is a billionaire and another is a guy who's building a small cabin to live in on his Social Security payments. No matter what their current life situation, it becomes obvious very quickly that problems are something all of us must face. The meetings are a great way to find fellowship with other people who can understand what you're going through, no matter how dark it is. I've shown up to this group feeling angry, frustrated, or hopeless and halfway through the meeting found that someone else was going through similar feelings.

Al-Anon (or one of the other Anonymous groups) is a dedicated support group that is there in a nonjudgmental way on days when you feel in control and, most helpfully, on days when you feel the lowest. Some of the topics that might be discussed in an Al-Anon meeting: excessive caretaking of another person, detaching with love, codependency, releasing the need to control, and self-blame. All of the topics encourage introspection and lead to deeper self-understanding.

I find "The Serenity Prayer," spoken at Al-Anon meetings, to be a calming reminder that the best approach to all of our problems is wisdom.

God grant me the serenity to accept the things I cannot change;
Courage to change the things I can;
And wisdom to know the difference.
—Reinhold Niebuhr

Making an effort to be around other people began slowly to dissolve the stigma I had felt about my depression. I had sequestered myself away for month after month, feeling ashamed of my inability to "snap out of it." I have pride and didn't want anyone to feel sorry for me. I was to learn later, through therapy, that a common reaction to depression is isolation. You feel so alone in your horrible pain that you keep to yourself. Unfortunately, we create our own prison, locking ourselves away, when what we need most is love, understanding of the disease, and interaction. This can only happen by finding ways to step out of our isolation.

One evening I was driving home from an Al-Anon meeting, after having hugged almost everyone in the group, when a memory came back to me that reminded me of the life-and-death necessity of giving and receiving affection. Early in my career as an RN, I was working my shift in the pediatrics ward. A little boy, who was small for his age, was admitted to the hospital suffering from malnutrition. His eyes were dull and he lay on the bed motionless, staring up at the ceiling. When I asked the attending physician what the child's diagnosis was, he showed me the words he had written on the boy's chart: "Failure to Thrive Syndrome." His parents were both drug addicts, and they had never held or cuddled him. They did not bond with their son and he was wasting away. My heart broke in a million pieces for this little guy. He was dying from a lack of human connection and love.

Human touch is as important to the body and soul as food and water. More and more people are coming to realize that having regular contact with others helps us to live happier, more satisfying, and even longer lives.

Dr. Dean Ornish's fascinating book, *Love and Survival,* is one of my personal favorites. For years he studied why human beings need each other. What he found is that isolation is more of a risk to the health of our hearts than smoking, obesity, and a sedentary lifestyle. Dean has been a friend for several decades now, and one time when he was at my farm he told me that anyone without significant friendships is two times more likely to die seven to ten years early than someone who has developed a close network of friends. Our brains are hardwired to connect with each other. It's his professional advice that we have at least seven to ten contacts with other people every single week.

According to the last Current Population Survey from the U.S. Census Bureau, 27 percent of Americans live alone. There's nothing wrong with that, unless it leaves you isolated and feeling like you have no community. It needs to be a priority to stay involved with other people, even when you don't feel like it. More than soothing loneliness, having a sense of connection to others has been shown to be a preventative approach for health issues like heart disease, ulcers, and possibly dementia, as it keeps our minds active.

Human touch soothes us. It activates the release of our love and compassion hormone, oxytocin. As Michelangelo already knew in the sixteenth century, "To touch can be to give life." Modern studies and science have proven his words to be true.

One of the most curative and healing occurrences for me, over the past two years, has been spending more time with Ashley. She perceived that I needed the security and stability that being in her presence provided for me. When we were together, Ashley would hold my hand. Anytime she was sitting beside me, she would put her arm around my shoulders. She would hug me "hello" and "goodbye" and say how much she loved me.

Another dependable comfort for me was having Larry continue with his daily morning routine, no matter what the night before had held for me. I could count on knowing that Larry would have the coffee made and be sitting at the kitchen table reading his scriptures. After taking the dogs outside and checking the horses, he would always give me the scoop on what had occurred in our "wild kingdom" overnight. Often his updates would bring a smile to my face.

One morning he returned to the house laughing. He had gone to feed our barn cats from the sealed plastic bin where he keeps their dry food, only to find that a raccoon had managed to pry it open, climb in, and gorge himself on so much cat food that he could only lie there staring up at Larry over his protruding belly. Having Larry so unwavering in his routine reminded me that life didn't have to be a daily struggle of emotional ups and downs, that it could also be enjoyable again.

Larry represented a steadfast flow of consistency and a calm manner in his approach to day-to-day life. This was healing for me. As my therapist, Diana, said to me, people with post-traumatic stress disorder are so familiar with feeling and perceiving drama both internally and externally that they tend unconsciously to look for more things to upset them. We have become so accustomed to the adrenaline rush that trauma has deposited in our nervous systems that we have become addicted to chronic chaos.

Acupuncture became my "go-to" therapy for calming down my nervous system. When I had hepatitis C, I tried every healing modality available because modern medicine had nothing to offer me. The treatment of hep C has advanced greatly since the early 1990s, but at that time I was on my own . . . once again.

I returned for acupuncture treatments to my favorite certified medical doctor, Dr. Xiao Mei Zhao. She was a bit shocked at my appearance, twenty pounds lighter, gaunt, and with barely any hair on my head. She was taken aback, but not discouraged. Chinese medicine has been used successfully to treat both acute and chronic illnesses for more then three thousand years. Dr. Zhao believes in it fully and has decades of knowledge about acupuncture stored in her brilliant mind. As she had explained to me, "If pain exists, either physical or mental, then your energy is trapped and stagnant. There is no free flow."

Acupuncture works on the healthy energy by the insertion of very thin needles along the body's meridians. The meridians are related to each of the main organs. It's a holistic approach that works with your own inner forces and immune system to cure what ails you. As I like to joke, "Just a little jab will do ya!"

After a few weekly treatments, Dr. Zhao consulted with me on my post-traumatic stress disorder. She said it was persistently stored in my system because I had gone so long without having it released. From her Eastern healing perspective, she told me, "The main treatment for depression always involves identifying and containing your memories and putting them in the right place." You can't be free of your negative memories, but they don't need to influence your day-to-day decisions or life anymore.

The "right place" is far away from your nervous system and stored in your brain under the category of history, a time that is gone and no longer needs to affect your current feelings.

I've found that acupuncture has been beneficial in helping me relax more fully. It eases my anxiety and I know it has helped me detox from some of the side effects of the unhelpful prescription drugs I was put on over the course of a year and a half. A good acupuncturist will listen fully to you and treat your worst symptoms first.

There are well-qualified acupuncturists even practicing in small towns now. You may be able to find one who can work on a sliding scale or might cut their rate if you buy in bulk, say 15 percent off five treatments. You can always ask.

The other form of healing touch that I began as a way to treat the stress of depression and anxiety was to have a massage every other week.

What my massage therapist helped me understand is that the sympathetic nervous system is overactivated when you have anxiety or depression or both. Our body's way of dealing with stress or perceived danger is the "fight-or-flight" reaction. Our heart rate increases and a surge in adrenaline courses through our system. Our blood flow goes to our limbs because our body believes it's time to run to escape danger. Our brains can't tell the difference between a real threat and a memory of a traumatic experience, which is why our bodies suffer with every memory of trauma. Massage therapy gives a boost to the parasympathetic system, which works in the opposite way of the sympathetic nervous system by lowering blood pressure, increasing overall blood flow, calming the digestive system, and soothing our pain receptors and nerves. It reminds you from the top of your head to the tip of your toes that you're a whole body, not just a head dragging a body around.

For myself, to relax completely, I need to feel that I don't have to converse with my massage therapist once I lie down on the massage table. It's important to let in the healing and that's hard to do if you feel obligated to hold up your end of a conversation.

I've actually asked massage therapists to please not say a word. It helps me not feel drained by their energy field.

My massage therapist, Kilie, has helped me tremendously over the last year and a half. At the beginning of our appointment, she listens intently to my current state of mind. She plays some soft music and stops talking completely until the massage is finished. She chooses an essential oil, like calming eucalyptus oil, to add to her massage oil based on how I described what I was feeling. The aromatherapy factor has its own healing effect. Practitioners of aromatherapy believe that the fragrance of the oil stimulates the part of the brain that controls our emotional memories. Depending on the fragrance used, the oil can be stimulating or relaxing. For example, peppermint can make you feel more alert, lemon oil produces a feeling of joy, lavender relaxes and helps you sleep, and smelling grapefruit oil helps to reduce the feeling of hunger.

Thanks to all of these different approaches to healing, as Larry noticed, I was improving day by day, with far fewer setback days. About once a week I would spiral downward into a feeling of hopelessness. On those days I would remember Diana's advice to make a list of pleasant activities and do at least one or two of them. On my list are things like: reading a science magazine, listening to music I love, spending time outside in our meditation garden, playing with the dogs, sorting photos, or organizing my kitchen cupboards and utensil drawers. The prescribed medications from Dr. Rosenbaum seemed to be leveling out the deepest lows and providing a platform from which to do more self-work with Diana through dialectical behavior therapy.

One afternoon, I spent a couple hours with Ashley at a mall. We wanted to pick up some yard games and toys for the kids who attend the family of choice Sunday picnics. We were having a fun mother-daughter time when my eyes landed on a Hello Kitty carrying case for pens, pencils, and crayons. A memory came back in full force of a time when having enough money to buy my own children toys was out of the question. I remembered how Ashley, at about age eight, picked up a Hello Kitty lunchbox when we had gone into a discount store for the bare necessities.

She carried it with her throughout the store, swinging it happily at her side.

When we got into the checkout line, I had to break the bad news to my little girl that she couldn't have the seven-dollar lunchbox. Seven dollars would buy two packages of lunch meat, canned soup, and vegetables, which would be two meals for all three of us. She didn't whine or beg or even shed a tear. She merely ran back to put it on the shelf where she had found it. I knew it was a big deal for her. I knew every other little girl in her class had a new lunchbox, while my girls carried their sandwiches in leftover brown bags.

With the painful memory came a tear that I wiped away quickly. I didn't want to ruin our afternoon. But once we got back to the car, I presented my adult daughter with the Hello Kitty carry case. I knew she no longer would want one, but I had to do it for both of us. Ashley smiled softly in recognition.

I told Larry about this story when I returned home. He nodded, but stayed silent. He is the girls' Pop and he loves them both as much as I do. Later that evening, Larry said, "I've got something I need to do. Mary will come over and watch TV with you. I won't be long."

I didn't know where he was planning to go; I only noticed the look of resolve on his face. He was on a mission.

Chapter 19
Every Ending Is a New Beginning

Wynonna's coming over for dinner tomorrow night," Larry said almost nonchalantly when he came home. He turned around and called for the dogs, to take them out one more time before bedtime.

"She hasn't come over in almost a year," I said, stunned. I followed Larry to the door. "What have you been up to?"

Larry took my hands in his. "I couldn't stand by and watch you be heartbroken anymore. Being estranged from Wy has played a big part in your depression. It's time for things to get better between you two."

I assumed Larry had probably shared with Wy quite a bit about what I had been going through. I also knew he was right.

The following evening I cooked Wy's favorite meal of chicken "Continental," a savory dish of browned chicken baked with seasoned rice, green Jell-O salad, asparagus, and hot rolls. When she arrived, we hugged warmly. We didn't talk about our relationship issues, because we needed to be in each other's presence for a while without turmoil. There was still a silent wall between us, but at least we were in the same room.

We had a pleasant evening as a family and I got to hear a lot about her upcoming tour. It pained my heart a little to know I wouldn't be a part of it, but I decided that I had to "radically accept" that she was now a successful solo act. Actually, she had been a hit solo act for years before our reuniting as the Judds for the Encore tour.

By the end of the evening, I was calm and had a deeper understanding of why our relationship has had its bumps and bruises. More than anyone else in my life, Wynonna had been with me through every trial and triumph that defined the person I became, both publicly and privately. From the time I was an eighteen-year-old new mother, through my divorce, abandonment, financial struggles, physical and mental assaults, heartbreaks, many relocations, educational quests, fears, and feats of courage, Wynonna was a witness to all of it. Then, when we teamed up to "sing for our supper," striving to be noticed and pay our dues in the music industry, we did it together, sometimes with wisdom but mostly by our bare wits. When you share a forty-five-foot-long tour bus as your home for most of a decade, there are no secrets. We knew everything about each other. We created shows, we wrote songs, we rehearsed, we argued, we laughed, we defended each other, we looked out for each other, and we cared deeply about our fans. Besides Ashley, there really was no one else who truly understood what it took for us to get where we were. The many awards we won were icing on a cake that was made with hard-earned ingredients. I was extremely proud of the career we built together. I didn't want the bond to be broken.

However, I am no longer that young woman, using every ounce of my natural determination and grit to make something of myself. I did, already. I need only to look around me to see what the sowing of my hard work over the decades has reaped. I didn't need to be afraid of abandonment and loss anymore. And Wynonna is no longer the talented teenager I needed to protect, push, and promote, to advise and assist with problems. She's an adult woman in her fifties, with grown children, a happy marriage, and at the peak of her creative journey as a solo artist. Even if I weren't her mother, I would say that Wynonna has one of the most captivating, soul-filled, world-class voices to ever grace a stage. I miss being with her, but I would never want her to miss out on accomplishing everything her talent deserves.

I know that now we each have a very different perspective of reality. They don't match up well. It takes extra effort for Wy to understand my reality and where I'm coming from, and for me to understand hers. Wy and I could not possibly be more different in our most elemental natures, with the exception of both being head-strong women. Being an "odd couple" onstage has always worked in our favor because the fans seemed to love the unpredictable banter and the contrast between mother and daughter, yet it isn't easy off-stage. Coming to understand and accept this has been a relief and has helped me to stop always wishing it could be different. I won't ever change her reality and the only thing that makes sense is for me to be clear about my own priorities and boundaries. I knew that I had to "radically accept" that concept, stop trying to defend myself, and stop asking her to justify her viewpoints. They are what they are. We are both right according to our own realities. Our own perception is our reality.

I have come to a place of self-forgiveness for the hundreds of mistakes I most likely made as a very young single mother who didn't have the resources to make great choices, had never experienced a mother's love, and who was always struggling to make sure we all had food on the table and clothing on our backs. I'm well aware Wy's and Ashley's growing-up years were not ideal, but they also held times of great joy and always love.

I hope someday both of my daughters will remember the good days as outweighing the bad. There is nothing I want more in the world than for my girls to be happy.

As Wy told Dan Rather on his show *The Big Interview* early in 2015, when he asked if the two of us talk regularly: "Our last tour was devastating. We don't talk much. It's going to take time. I think because I'm a mom right now. And dealing with teenagers—and paybacks are hell. I miss her."

*   *   *

After this dinner with Wynonna, I felt my own mother on my mind, and I began thinking of her constantly, picturing her in that nursing home in Kentucky. She had spent her life in the house I grew up in, the one my parents bought from my Judd grandparents, Ogden and Sally Judd, when I was four years old. It had become her avocation, her one true love. She was always redecorating: painting the walls and buying new furniture and housewares. She even entertained in the house after her second marriage. Now, everyone's gone, her second husband having passed away years ago, and she's in a nursing home. She knows the house, her masterpiece, has been sold. She can no longer amaze people with her cooking talents. She has to eat institutional food and live in a "home" with other people who are all strangers to her. The pendulum of my emotions continues to swing between sadness, pity, anger toward her, and, still, love for my mother.

In my first book, *Love Can Build a Bridge,* I painted a picture of Mother as far more maternal than she ever was. I think I wrote it that way to gain her approval and give her some status in the community of Ashland. I wanted to protect and defend her, because her life was never easy.

Defending her was something I did from my earliest years. When I was growing up, wearing a hat to church was the popular fashion. Mother worked in the nursery every Sunday, never sitting in with the congregation with us. She only had three dresses, so I figured that she didn't want others to notice. One Sunday, a well-to-do snooty country club–type woman stopped me in the hallway before the service and said, "I never see your mother wearing a hat." It bothered me deeply that she was pointing this out, loud enough for others to hear. After thinking quickly on my feet I responded equally loudly, "She doesn't wear a hat, because she's afraid your kids will knock it off." The truth was, my mom didn't own a hat.

My mother spent so many years feeling both anonymous and humiliated about her difficult life that it wasn't hard to understand how she became bitter. But even when things went her way, she was unable to be happy. She remained negative, judgmental, and harsh in her opinions of others.

I knew how much she longed to be respected and admired. I used my name and endorsement in the late 1990s to get her elected as city commissioner, which was a point of great pride for her. She had a bit of power and could use her natural intelligence. When her term was up she wasn't reelected because, by then, people had come to know her. She would say things that got her in trouble. The night she lost her bid for re-election she called me crying, "I don't know what happened."

A number of years ago, when phones still had answering machines with cassette tapes for messages, I came home to find a rare phone message from Mother, who almost never called me. On the tape, she complimented me: "I know I don't say this enough, dear, but I'm very proud of you. You make people feel good. You treat me so well. Thank you for sending me money." I still have that cassette tape because I knew it might be the only time I ever heard affectionate words from my mother.

When I began feeling more emotionally stable, I thought it might be an opportune time to connect with Mother. I also wanted to prove to myself that I could now cope with highly emotional situations. Larry and I drove the six hours to Ashland to take her out shopping to Kroger for food and supplies for her room at the nursing home. We drove her through Central Park, where my siblings and I played as kids, and from one end of town to the other so she could look at everything she wanted to see. Then we pulled into the Wendy's drive-through for a chocolate Frosty, which is one of her favorite treats.

At the end of the day we took her to dinner at her favorite restaurant, the Chimney Corner. People she knew stopped by our table to chat. She was in a conversational mood and began talking with us about family history. She lamented how dysfunctional the Judds had been and how much it had affected her on a daily basis.

I decided to take a big chance and reveal to Mother what the last thirty months of my life had been like. I put my hands on the table, hoping she might reach across and touch me. After I finished telling her, she slowly dropped her eyes to her plate as if she was taking in what I had said, then picked up her fork and ate her last two bites of chicken. She looked up at me with a dismissive glance and asked, "Shall we see what's on the dessert bar?"

And that was that. Larry couldn't believe her coldness to me. He put his arm around me and pulled me into his chest. When we took her back to her room, I stopped and turned at the door as Larry and I were leaving and said, "I love you, Mother."

She shrugged and answered, "Love ya." Then, as I smiled, she sternly warned me, "Don't talk about our family."

I have closed the door for good on any wishful thinking I once held tight that she might be capable of motherly compassion. It's simply too late. On her table in her nursing home are a few photos of family, but in the most prominent place is the photo of her beaming next to Jack Nicholson that I took after the Grammy Awards. It's still a source of satisfaction for her and she loves when people ask her about meeting him. She's eighty-nine years old now and I will continue to visit her. I want her final years to be comfortable, no matter what our relationship can never become.

I found a lovely apartment close to where I live in Tennessee, with large windows and a huge veranda. It was handy to a grocery store, shops, and good restaurants. She could also order anything she wanted and have it delivered. I put down a deposit and had it painted her favorite colors. I arranged to have furniture delivered and I called Mother to tell her that I knew how badly she wanted to be out of the nursing home and I had arranged a solution.

She refused the gift. She didn't want to leave. She wanted to remain in the gray and dreary town of Ashland, steeping in her memories of a life gone sour.

* * *

As I focused in on my dialectical behavior therapy, Diana helped me to recognize that I was starting to think and react in a more healthy way. I began to extend myself a bit more with each passing day, and the challenges I faced didn't make me feel as hopeless thanks to my

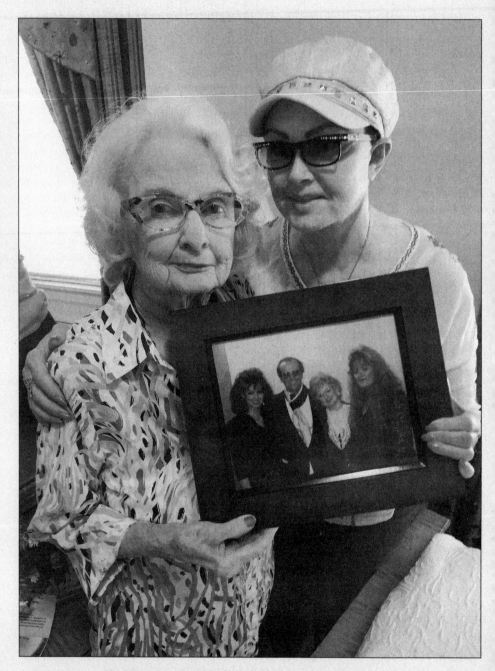

*My mother, September 2016, with her treasured photo of posing with
actor, Jack Nicholson, backstage at the Grammy awards.*

new skills at regulating my emotions which brought a welcome shift, uplifting my down-in-the-dumps perspective. However, there were still triggers that could set off a depressive spiral or overwhelmingly strong anxiety. For example, I was in the waiting room of a doctor's office, and feeling pretty good, when "Clair de Lune" was piped in over the speakers. I was instantly overcome by a profound anxiety. I had to leave the building and go outside into the sunshine. I found myself leaning against the brick wall next to a couple of employees who had stepped outside to smoke. I began to sob uncontrollably.

I had a distinct sad memory of an interaction with my father from when I was seventeen and had found out I was pregnant but hadn't told anyone yet. My piano teacher had called the house to find out why I had skipped two weeks of lessons. I had been memorizing "Clair de Lune" to play at the next recital when my life changed permanently with my unexpected pregnancy. Previously, I had never missed a lesson. Playing piano was one of the few joys of my childhood and I would even put on my Sunday dress at home, place a lighted candle on the piano top, and open the windows to serenade the neighbors as I practiced.

Daddy had heard that the teacher said, "Naomi could be a great classical pianist, but I can't get her to practice anymore. It's a shame if she gives it up now."

Daddy confronted me by complaining, "I work like a damn brute to come up with the dollar fifty a week for you to have those piano lessons." The disappointed look on his face crushed me, but more than that, it was the first time I had ever heard Daddy use a swear word. At age seventeen, it felt like nothing would ever be okay again. Hearing "Clair de Lune" triggered the same feeling of being a failure because I couldn't overcome my depression and anxiety.

I told Diana of my emotional reaction at the piped-in music in a waiting room. I expressed my fear of being caught unexpectedly in public having an overwhelming response, because my emotions felt so unpredictable.

Diana reminded me, "How many public places have you been in your life without any issues? How many hotel lobbies, waiting rooms, movie theaters, lecture halls, and restaurants? You've been fine many, many more times than times when you've had an issue. Right?"

I had to admit she had a good point.

She smiled and then offered me this piece of advice: "When you feel weak, anxious, or frightened, say this to yourself: 'I'm Naomi Freakin' Judd and I've got this.'"

One afternoon, I was with four girlfriends in a small café. We were all catching up when suddenly I could feel a rising panic in me. My heart started to race and my palms became sweaty. I wasn't sure what had happened, but I wanted to get up and go home immediately. My girlfriends gathered around me with concern. I knew that it wouldn't help me to give in to the anxiety. Larry was out at a rehearsal and I really didn't want to be alone. I wanted to be around my friends. I applied the mindfulness technique I had learned at Promises and started taking long, slow breaths. I told myself: Look around. You're in the village. You're at a café you've been to many times. You are safe. You are with friends you love.

I looked at what was right there in my environment. What was the design on Helen's blouse? How many beads were on Rachel's bracelet? Then I started thinking of what I liked the most about each of my friends. Soon the distraction helped my overactive amygdala settle down. For other people, successfully getting past a panic attack in this manner might seem trivial, but for people who have them, we know we just reached the summit of Mount Everest. No easy feat, but I'm Naomi Freakin' Judd, and I've got this.

I began to read again. I wanted a different perspective on the idea that I would be forever stained with the genetic legacy of mental illness passed down to me.

My friend of twenty-five years, Dr. Francis Collins, one of the world's leading genetic scientists, and I have spent quite a bit of time talking about his work. One evening during his visit to our farm, I told him I was curious about what he knew about our inheritable predispositions in our genes and if they are set in stone or can be changed or influenced. He explained to me the theory of epigenetics, where a gene can be altered through environmental factors, both in negative and positive ways.

New findings are providing evidence of transgenerational epigenetic inheritance and that the environment can affect an individual's genes, which can be passed on to the next generation. This left me to contemplate that if genetics could predispose a person to a 50 percent higher risk of alcoholism, as has been proven, could it also work for optimism? Could qualities like gratitude, good intentions, being nurturing, and having a positive attitude change the structure of our genes and be passed down to the next generation, too?

Out of curiosity, I explored this subject further, and found the work of Bruce Lipton (*The Biology of Belief*), a research scientist with radical ideas about how our genes can be influenced. His theory is that while we are predisposed genetically to have certain abilities, strengths, weaknesses, and diseases, including depression, these attributes are not necessarily our fate through heredity. Through his studies and research he noted that our environment and our perceptions of our circumstances equally influence our cells. Genes are not destiny after all. It's very possible, and is being proven more and more through research all the time, that the mind can control matter at least as much as matter controls our minds. What fabulous news, especially for someone, like me, with mental illness in the family.

According to epigenetic research, one-third of our genetic makeup is controlled by heredity, but the other two-thirds are influenced by our environment and personal choices. So perhaps more of my biology was in my control than I thought. Maybe I was less doomed than the original recipe of my DNA was predicting. Put simply, it seems that if we can rethink and release any long-held beliefs that we are doomed to be sick or weak or are stuck with a batch of bad genes handed down from mom and pop, then we can change the subconscious mind and our genes to help us heal. But we have to replace the bombardment of negative beliefs with positive thoughts and conscious actions.

Dr. Rosenbaum and I would talk by phone. He even gave me his cell phone number. Like a broken record, in every phone call he would remind me about the importance of exercise. I understand why. If I lie on the couch, I get into trouble. My thoughts spiral into dark and hopeless places. When you exercise you are active, and so are your thoughts. There is inarguable proof now that exercise produces endorphins, which trigger a positive feeling in the body. It's not always easy to feel like exercising, especially when you are in emotional pain. What I found the most helpful is to have someone I could look forward to seeing while I exercise.

My Pilates instructor, Tara, is more than an instructor. She's a healer for me. Every session with her starts and ends with hugs, support, and words of inspiration.

Pilates was developed for maintaining flexibility and strength in your core muscles, like your abdomen. Even on days when I don't feel like going, I know that I will leave feeling dramatically better. On other days, I take walks with my dogs as my form of exercise. That is therapeutic as well. It makes my dogs happy and that makes me feel happier. I've found that any type of movement gives me a better chance of improving than doing nothing. Larry and I even signed up for a line-dancing class with several friends. The music, the movement, and the laughter have healing powers.

I understand completely how exercise may seem overwhelming if you're depressed. On my worst days, Ashley would have to coax me fifty feet to the old oak tree in my yard. But even that amount of movement would change my perspective.

One benefit of having lost about twenty pounds from not being able to eat much was that I could wear some fun clothes. One weekend I called my grandson, Elijah, and said, "The Rolling Stones are in Nashville. My manager has third-row seats for you and Haley and me. Let's go!" I bought a fringe skirt, donned one of my show wigs, did my makeup, and off we went. We had an absolute blast. Elijah and Haley were blown away watching Mick Jagger strut defiantly across the stage at seventy-one years old. Seeing his ageless energy made me feel hopeful. I danced for the entire two and a half hours of the concert.

When I returned home, Larry was watching the late night news and I stopped in my tracks when I saw footage from the concert. The camera zoomed in on me, my arms raised in the air, cheering, whooping, and hollering. I heard the news anchor report, "Our own Naomi Judd was at the concert tonight, dancing away down front."

I was feeling very happy about it all. I'm Naomi Freakin' Judd, and I've got this.

Chapter 20

The Toothpaste Is Out
of the Tube

*"Make every effort to change things you do not like. If
you cannot make a change, change the way you have been
thinking. You might find a new solution."*
—MAYA ANGELOU

M aya Angelou was my solution to finding a maternal role
model. She mothered me for years because my own mother
didn't know how. She became my spiritual mother.

The first time I visited her comfortable home in North Carolina,
I was nervous about meeting this venerated wise woman.

In her book *I Know Why the Caged Bird Sings*, Maya wrote how,
during her childhood, the big treat on Christmas Day was to enjoy
a can of Dole pineapple. I dared to bake her a homemade pineapple
upside-down cake, which delighted her. Maya washed it down with a
glass of Johnnie Walker Red, her lunchtime drink of choice, proving
her preferences were always true to the South.

Over the years we would sit in her beautifully planted colorful
garden and talk about all manner of things. Her slowly enunciated
speech enraptured me and I would take in her wise advice to my
questions about the complications of family relationships.

When the sun would spill over to where we were lounging, she would put up her parasol. She would admonish me that I should always carry a parasol to protect my "alabaster porcelain skin" from the sun's harmful rays.

The last time we parted, I teasingly warned her that on my next visit I was going to bring her a puppy. Without missing a beat, Maya snapped back, "Fine, I will have another daughter waiting for you."

A year after she passed away, a package arrived from her estate. It was the white lace parasol she used while meditating in that garden. Now I can sit in my own garden, under this precious keepsake, replaying our laughter and conversations.

This magical woman lived her life with deep meaning until the very end. It was the most important example she could bequeath to following generations.

I was ready to radically accept that my prior purpose in life, of touring and performing for millions of people, was over. It was incredibly painful to release it. But it hurt less than emotionally holding on to a history that couldn't be repeated. I had to find a new purpose. As soon as my pain became overwhelming, I loosened my grip on the past and my future began to knock on my door. My motto became, Acknowledge. Allow. Accept.

I needed to dive into something that held great meaning for me, so I became a board member of the American Humane Association. Many people think the AHA is about cats and dogs, but it's much more. The AHA is the dedicated group that helped to finally outlaw the use of elephants in the circus and send them to sanctuaries. They also are working on protecting the gentle manatees in Florida that are injured and killed by boat propellers and jet-skis. You can also find the AHA on every movie and television set where they are using animals. If you watch a stunt horse falling in a movie, you don't have to worry. We are there overseeing that it's not hurt. We watch over creatures, both great and small, which need protection, since they have no voice.

I've been invited to Florida with the AHA on a mission to reunite military bomb-sniffing dogs with the soldiers who were partnered with them. These beloved German shepherd dogs were responsible for saving between 100 and 170 American lives each day during the height of the Iraq War. They have been specifically trained to sniff out bombs or IED explosives underground. The dogs also supply comfort and solace to our service people who are in volatile and anxiety-filled situations.

I had the privilege of meeting five injured Marines who had been sent home from Fallujah, Iraq, within the past year. The men not only suffered the effects of post-traumatic stress disorder from coming under fire; they were also not healing well from their emotional injuries. The doctors said one of the reasons they weren't getting better was that they had been in inner turmoil about the unknown fate of their service dogs since the time of the blasts that injured them.

The American Humane Association located all five dogs and had them shipped back to the States to be reunited with their human soldiers in Florida. It was a difficult process, since the dogs are considered property of the military; their training is an $85,000 investment. Some of the dogs had been relocated within the army but were not faring well separated from their original human partners.

The reunion of a soldier and his K-9 and the unbridled joy and healing it brought was enough to light my fire of purpose. I went to work making changes. I refused to accept that these war hero dogs had no medical coverage. I spent several days on Capitol Hill with the AHA president, Robin Ganzert, speaking to many of our representatives to encourage them to pass a law that would allow these hero war dogs to get full veterinary coverage once they return to the United States. In addition, any dog whose soldier is killed in the line of duty should eventually come home to that hero's family. It's been an education, helping to pass legislation in Congress, but I've been invigorated by the challenge. Who better to give my time and energy to than our American heroes, including the four-legged ones? I plan to stay active in this cause to make sure our hero dogs are reunited with their hero service person.

In addition, I am working on getting two police dogs for the use of the city where I live. I was infuriated to learn that one of our officers' K-9s had been shot and killed by the perpetrator in a bank robbery. The criminal was only charged with a misdemeanor in killing the dog. Considering the cost of training these magnificent loyal dogs, not to mention their intrinsic worth as our fellow creatures, I fought to get harming a service dog changed under Tennessee law from a misdemeanor to a felony. They also deserve a full burial ceremony.

A dog doesn't have to be on a battlefield or at a crime location to be a hero. In 2016, *People* magazine published a special collector's edition, "American Heroes," featuring a yellow Lab named Bella. She is a service dog and a hero to her owner, a young woman who has suffered paralyzing panic attacks for years, and who had been hospitalized for both depression and anxiety. She was struggling to live on her own when Bella was brought into her life. This beautiful canine companion had been trained to notice rising anxiety in a human and supply him or her with comfort and distraction. Because of Bella, the young woman is able to live independently, even though she still faces her mental illnesses daily.

I almost always travel with my small dog, Bijou. My psychiatrist gave me a document stating that Bijou is necessary for my emotional wellbeing. She wears a little vest to identify her as a service dog. The emotional support and the comfort Bijou brings me is incalculable. My dogs are my best friends and they have carried me through my darkest days.

One afternoon, Larry found me upstairs in the bedroom, staring out the window at the breathtaking countryside, blooming with summertime life. He sat on the arm of my chair and put his arm around my shoulder, pulling me toward him.

"I need to say this. I am concerned that you don't attend church. The only time you pray is over supper," Larry said.

I couldn't understand why my husband was confronting me with this now, with all that I had been through.

"I've never stopped praying for you," he continued. "Honey, there is a God. Believing in something bigger than your problems is how you're going to get through all of this. There is a Supreme Being, a Divine Intelligence, a love that created the universe and is much more than our imagination can comprehend. God is there and loves you unconditionally."

I knew he was right. God wasn't the one who gave me depression or made it seem difficult or unfair. He had granted me free will to make my own choices. Maybe the time had come to "radically accept" that I couldn't know the reason why I had this brain disease, at least for now. I was willing to begin practicing my belief in a Divine Creator.

Later that night I had a life-altering revelation. It came to me when I was awakened with a panic attack. I felt a sense of protection, like a comforting presence, come into the room.

I've always been a woman who needed to reconcile God and science to fully commit and surrender in faith. I've come to understand that the two aren't mutually exclusive. Science tells us how; faith tells us why. The next day I began to read *The Hidden Face of God*, by the brilliant physicist Gerald Schroeder. He wrote: "A single consciousness, an all-encompassing wisdom, pervades the universe. The discoveries of science, those that search the quantum nature of sub-atomic matter, those that explore the molecular complexity of biology, and those that probe the brain/mind interface, have moved us to the brink of a startling realization: all existence is the expression of this wisdom."

Are we each a part of that universal wisdom? If what Gerald Schroeder has concluded through research is true, then we must be.

As they say in the twelve-step program, this is "God as I understand God."

With faith, I can see the wisdom of God now using me to help other people, even if it's just by sharing my most vulnerable and painful times so others feel less alone. By doing this, I don't feel so alone anymore. An unseen presence is guiding and comforting me.

Larry encouraged me to return to an idea that had bloomed in my mind when I was out on the Encore tour. During the meet-and-greets after the shows, fans would often share their troubles and mention how our music would help them through. Music is healing for me, as well. I had mentioned to Larry late one night, as our tour bus rumbled along to the next city, that it might be a gift to suffering people to record a CD that contained calming music along with uplifting quotes and scriptures. We could leave a part of ourselves to future generations. Now it seemed was the perfect time to follow through on this new idea, "Comforting Words & Music."

Larry and I began creating peaceful music at our home recording studio, because I wanted to make sure it was perfect. I had studied psychoacoustics, which is the science behind how music affects brain wave activity. We all recognize how music affects our moods. Rap and hip-hop music makes me feel hyper and jittery. Subtle instrumental music with sounds from nature calms me.

I gathered up some of my favorite inspirational sayings and Bible verses and we recorded them. Then Larry recorded the most lovely music underneath the words.

I sent the first copy, hot off the press, to my friend, the beautiful country singer Joey Feek. She had been diagnosed with recurring stage 4 cervical cancer, which had now spread. Joey had decided to give up on medical treatment, which wasn't working anymore. She had moved to Indiana to be closer to family, with her husband and singing partner, Rory, and their darling baby girl, a special needs child. Joey wanted to remain as lucid as possible and enjoy the time she had left with Rory and her baby, though her hundreds of thousands of fans, including me, never stopped praying for a miracle. Since I wouldn't be able to travel to Indiana to see her, I sent her a copy of the CD and a letter. About a week later, Rory called to say that Joey listened to the CD, on repeat, all day long. I was deeply moved and grateful that it could bring her comfort in her final weeks. It was exactly what I hoped this special music could do for others.

If I can bring any comfort or hope to you, too, that would give my writing this book the greatest meaning. I may still struggle, but I no longer suffer. I want to share some of the insights I have gained and techniques I have used almost every day:

• **If you become ill with an emotional illness, have a loved one help you plan your course of treatment.** You'll need a trusted ear and eye to help you watch over your condition until you feel more stable and have clarity. Don't make big decisions while you're in a depressed state. This person can also help you find a therapy that will help you. Many cities and counties have free health clinics that include mental health. There are also therapists who work on a sliding scale. Group therapy is a more low-cost way to receive the benefit of a therapist and also provides the support of other people who struggle with mental illness.

Consider attending one of the many twelve-step groups going on in most cities in the United States. If you live in a rural area, you can now attend meetings by Skype. There are no permanent or appointed leaders or professional therapists in the twelve-step groups and there is no cost to attend. Often the best therapy is being able to talk about what you're going through, out loud, with a group of people who understand and support each other's efforts to be well. There are now twelve-step programs and meetings for almost every issue for which depression and anxiety might be the cause or a side effect. There are meetings for gamblers, survivors of incest, hepatitis C, narcotics, and nicotine cravings. There are meeting for overeaters and sex addicts, those with eating disorders, and workaholics. There are even groups called Emotions Anonymous, whose purpose is to help people understand and unravel their destructive emotions and lead more manageable lives. Your scariest and most private fears are shared by thousands of other people. When you're ready to talk about your fear, you're no longer alone anymore.

There is great solace in being around others who truly understand what it's like to be depressed or suffer panic attacks. Some universities and colleges even offer free clinics for psychological services where you can have sessions with their doctors and social workers in training. If you feel you can't discuss needing help with a friend or family member, then you can call 211. In almost every part of the country, dialing 211 will connect you to a caring listener who can direct you to social programs or emergency shelters and resources. Know the number for the suicide hotline in your state. Find it online at suicide.org. If you feel at your limit, please pick up the phone and call.

• **If you live in a cloudy part of the country, get some Happy Lights**. Many of us are affected by seasonal affective disorder. These large tabletop lamps provide full-spectrum light, which is comparable to sunlight. They help to regulate the circadian cycle of a twenty-four-hour day. On dreary weather days, I keep two on my kitchen table.

Our bodies make vitamin D through our skin when it has sunlight exposure. Insufficient levels of vitamin D are linked to clinical depression. Vitamin D supplements are inexpensive and easy to find. If you know you're not getting sunlight, ask your doctor about the appropriate dose. A simple blood test can determine if you need the supplement.

Also, the barometric pressure can influence how you feel, contributing to headaches, even migraines. It affects me and a number of my friends, as well.

• **Some people are finding relief from depression with a method of treatment called transcranial magnetic stimulation**. It doesn't produce seizures like electroconvulsive therapy, but seems to be successful for some in the same way. A magnetic coil is placed near your head and produces small electric currents in the region of the brain right under the coil. Evidence is suggesting that it's useful for people

with treatment-resistant depression and doesn't have the side effects
that electroconvulsive therapy might produce. I tried it for a number
of sessions, but the severity of my depression, along with overwhelming anxiety and panic, made it less effective for me, which is why Dr.
Rosenbaum suggested the ECT treatments in my case. That doesn't
mean it wouldn't be something worthwhile for you. I'm putting it on
the list because I think it holds promise for many.

• **Start now to write in a journal about your self-identity.** How
would you like to be known in the future? If one part of your life is
over (mom to little kids, employee, beauty, health, youth, etc.), then
how do you perceive the next phase of your life? Dream big.

• **Meditate.** I know it's hard to quiet your mind, but sit for ten minutes every day and give it a go. I sit upstairs in an armchair and look
out the window at nature. I try to focus on being totally present, not
thinking of the past or the future. It gives your brain a break and
relaxes your nervous system. There are hundreds of different meditation methods. You can find them online, on YouTube, or at the
library.

• **Take a college or adult education class.** Reignite your passions and find a course that interests you. I have a friend, Cherrie,
who takes a photography class at a technical college. She met new
people with a similar interest and they go on photography outings
together.

Vanderbilt University in Nashville offers classes for people over
age fifty for only twenty-five dollars. I've taken many: physics, art,
literature, anthropology, forensics, and creative writing. It motivates
me to get dressed up, out of the house, and into the world, and get

my brain into gear. Look into Osher Lifelong Learning Institutes. They have topics for every taste.

Find out about seminars or lectures you can attend at local community centers, art museums, libraries, hospitals, churches, and colleges. Your local weekly newspapers and magazines usually list these events. Many of them are free or offered at a low cost. It's a relief to the brain to learn something new, instead of recycling the same old thought patterns. I updated my ability to perform CPR at our local hospital. You can arrange to have a CPR instruction lesson with a group of your friends.

If it feels overwhelming to you to be around a roomful of people, begin with only one other person. Offer to babysit and hold and nurture someone else's child. Or volunteer to teach a child to read or tutor them in any subject. I believe our nation's children are starved for human touch and interaction. Too often, I see parents who depend on an iPad to keep their children occupied, while they are absorbed in their own electronic activities. Parenting can be exhausting and the need for a few hours of peace is understandable. But, in the long run, are we teaching kids that machines matter more than people?

• **Follow a sports team.** Get over-the-top enthusiastic about them. Meet up with other fans and cheer. I follow the University of Kentucky basketball team. Ashley has been a fervent longtime fan and it's such a kick to be around her. I'll wear blue and white and get loud and crazy over basketball. It's fun and a great way to scream and holler without hurting anyone's feelings.

• **Attend live music concerts.** Various studies have reported that playing or listening to music relieves persistent pain, both physical and emotional. Most churches have choirs or times when they practice and that are open to the public. Check out the music programs in your city; perhaps a town band is playing at your local park or choirs are performing for a special event, especially during the holidays, when many people struggle with depression. Colleges often offer open recitals by their music program students, free of charge. Larry and I enjoy our local bluegrass music.

• **Change up your day.** Try putting some new activity in your routine. Even a minor change can give you a fresh perspective. Take your magazine or newspaper and go for breakfast in a local diner. Chat with the waitstaff or other customers. Shop in a different grocery store from where you usually go. Wear clothes you've been "saving" for good. Get a new coffee or tea mug. Go for a manicure and choose a color you've never worn!

• **Volunteer for the Red Cross or at a homeless shelter.** Build a house with Habitat for Humanity. Help out at a Boys and Girls Club. Be a library or hospital volunteer. Giving to others gets you out of obsessing about your own problems. Find a cause. Make it yours.

This was the most powerful antidote for my depression. Watching out for animals is my passion. Besides working with the American Humane Association, I am assisting in the effort to get puppy mills closed down by getting city ordinances changed. This has been so rewarding for me that it's beyond description. We have to work under the radar so the puppy mill owners don't move or hide the dogs, so you'll have to ask your veterinarian or your local chapter of the Humane Society for more information.

Our brains need to rest from trying to solve our personal daily problems and issues. The best way to let your mind rest and also be productive is to be of service to someone else. You may find that you have a much better perspective on someone else's problems than you have on your own. My personal motto: Service is the work of the soul. I believe we are here to grow in wisdom and love and to be of service.

• **Exercise in any way you can.** A ten-minute walk; yoga; kickboxing; Pilates. Plant a garden. Decide to walk to the grocery store and back, instead of driving. Throw the ball for your dog. When the weather is gloomy, I drive to our local mall. I park at one end and walk the length of the mall and back. The brightly colored store windows lift my mood and help make the exercising easier.

• **If you don't have a pet, adopt a dog or cat.** Please, don't buy one at a pet store. Go to a shelter. You will bring home unconditional love. If you live somewhere you can't have a pet, then offer to walk a neighbor's dog. Or go to your local pet shelter and give some love to the abandoned animals. You can find where shelters are located on the internet. We always need volunteers.

• **Forgive yourself.** Being angry with yourself, or feeling shame or guilt for your depression or anxiety, will only take you further down. You didn't create your mental illness, so it's pointless to be self-critical about it. I can't emphasize this enough. It's a disease of the brain.

Start to respect yourself. You deserve it. You'll get better and look back on this time and feel proud of your progress. Wash the negative self-talk out of your mind with positive affirmations.

• **Write down the things that you'd like to hear and say them to yourself.**

My most difficult time of the day in battling depression is the morning. I have a routine I follow. I step out into my back yard and take a few deep breaths. I look around and notice what is growing. Then, when I take my medicine, I say a prayer of gratitude that they are working and supplying my brain with what it needs. One of the most famous affirmations was created more than a century ago by a French psychologist and pharmacist Émile Coué, who would tell patients to take their medication and say, "Every day, in every way, I'm getting better and better." He discovered that his patients recovered more rapidly if they repeated this mantra. Or choose an affirmation of your own, something simple, like "I'm relaxed," or "I am strong and stable." Repeat it to yourself as often as you can in the beginning. You can record your own voice saying your affirmations and listen to it while you cook or clean or go for a walk. Your brain will begin to accept and believe it.

I was at an airport recently, when a man approached me to ask if I would pray with him. He was attending his daughter's wedding and said, worriedly, "I'm getting the flu. Will you pray for me?" I replied, "Heck, no!" He gave me a puzzled look, so I explained. "Listen to what you said out loud, that you're getting the flu. Now, if you'd like to pray 'Thank you, God, that my immune system is strong and keeping me healthy' then I can do that. Pray the answer, never the problem."

Two of the pioneers of mind-body healing are Dr. Mona Lisa Schulz and Louise Hay. They have great books full of positive affirmations on health, healing, confidence, and finances that you can use if you can't think of your own. Both have audio books and printed books, and you can find them at your local library. You can find their affirmations at www.HayHouse.com. Louise Hay, who looks like a million bucks, is ninety years old, still lectures around the country, and has a radio and publishing business, so she's walking proof of the power of affirmations.

*   *   *

Every minute about one million of your cells die, replaced by an equal number of new cells. Perhaps because of heredity you have cells that bring depression or anxiety. They are on their way out. Every single molecule in your brain is replaced every two months. Now is the time to give yourself a psycho-spiritual makeover. Positive beliefs, prayer, visualizations of happy times, being in nature, gratitude, humor, exercise, rest, loving social networks, acts of kindness, goals, a sense of purpose—all have a powerful effect on all the major physical and mental systems of your body. We each have happy genes just waiting to express their potential. I know that it's difficult to believe, especially when you are in so much pain and you just want the pain to stop. You have to find some reason to stay alive through the darkest days, even if it's something simple.

All twenty-nine people who survived a suicide attempt from the Golden Gate Bridge said that they regretted their decision to kill themselves as soon as they jumped. All twenty-nine!

The therapeutic advice that has helped me the most is the concept of radical acceptance. Accept where you are right now. Once you have dealt with your subconscious issues or buried traumas, don't stay there and ruminate. You don't want to be a wound addict. Don't marinate in your problems. Don't spend time wishing it were different. For now, it's not. But it can be. Move forward from that place. It's a slow process, not a miraculous healing. You'll have times where you feel it's going to be okay and times where you still feel little hope. Accept that instead of letting it frighten you. The situation will change. Change is the true nature of life. Inch forward. Check your thoughts. Give yourself a way to think differently by making a change, even one that is imperceptible to others.

Don't isolate yourself. Reach out. I can't express how important it is to have social connection. You won't have to reach very far to

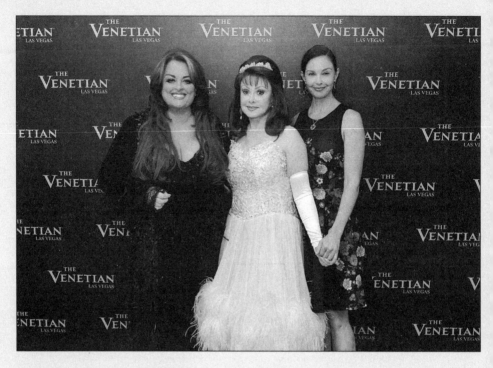

The finale at the Venetian Theatre in Las Vegas with the " jewels" in my crown.

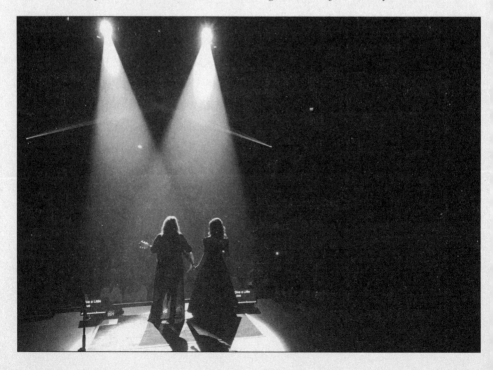

find someone who feels the way you do, has survived, and can help you to survive as well. And radical acceptance can come with helpful surprises you might never expect.

It seemed as if once I had radically accepted that my days onstage were over and I had fully involved myself in other purposeful pursuits for my future, out of the blue the phone rang.

My manager was calling to say that the Venetian in Las Vegas was asking Wynonna and me to reunite for a string of concert dates in October and November of 2015 in their elegant Venetian Theatre. It had been four years since Wynonna and I had performed a concert together.

I was thrilled to have the opportunity and immediately asked if Wynonna had accepted the invitation. She had. It moved me that she told the press, "I looked at this as an incredible chance to celebrate my Mom . . . to honor the roots that gave me the wings to fly."

Never say never. Suddenly my days were once again full to the brim with vocal training, rehearsals, finding stage gowns and shoes, and press opportunities. We named our concert "Girls Night Out," which was one of our number one singles from 1985. Here we were, thirty years later, still selling thousands of tickets. I couldn't wait to see the familiar smiling faces of all the fans once more.

Larry and I rented a condo in Vegas for the months of October and November and looked forward to being in the "Entertainment Capital of the World." It was like a honeymoon for us. After all Larry had gone through for my sake in taking care of me, he deserved a change of scenery and some fun at the casinos.

On the day of our press interviews in Las Vegas, Wynonna and I fell into step with each other onstage and had a good time answering questions. Wynonna was wearing her signature black and I decided to dress up in a forty-dollar dress I found in a vintage shop. It was a cream-colored floor-length satin gown with a ring of ostrich-sized white feathers surrounding the neckline. Of course, I had to top it off with a tiara in my hair, because more is more when it comes to bling.

Robin Leach, the well-known host of the onetime hit TV show *Lifestyles of the Rich and Famous*, now resides in Vegas and writes a column for the *Las Vegas Review Journal*. At a press conference held at noon he questioned me about wearing such an elaborate gown. When I asked him if he liked it, he replied that it was "hideous."

I shrugged it off, but Wynonna took Robin to the mat for his insensitive description. It evoked a clear remembrance of the mother-daughter team from thirty years ago, supporting and defending one another. When we took a break Wynonna went to find Robin and told him, "She's my mom. If she wants to show up in spandex and a tube top . . . go, girl." She insisted that Robin owed me an apology and he good-naturedly agreed.

Later, in typical Wy reasoning and humor, she told me, "He hurt your feelings and I'm not going to let that happen. If anyone's going to hurt your feelings, it'll be me."

This confirmed for me that our bond may have bent over time, but it still wasn't broken.

The staff and the show crew at the Venetian treated us like royalty and their professionalism was obvious in everything they did, matching the quality of the gorgeous theater. I even had a couple of Chippendale dancers join me onstage for a comedy bit, rising up through the stage floor on a platform.

When I stepped back onstage for the first show, I was overjoyed and moved to tears simultaneously. I had come full circle and was back home again. Performing is in my blood, whether it's acting on TV, in a movie, or entertaining an audience during a speaking engagement. Communicating with others is in my soul. I savor every second of these opportunities.

While going over the list of songs in Vegas, everyone unequivocally agreed that one of them should be "River of Time." I wrote this song in 1988, before my diagnosis with hepatitis C and long before I experienced severe depression. Songs take on different meaning as you progress through the stages of life and this one now held a more profound significance than ever before.

It was a thrill to be reunited with my daughter onstage, and it meant the world to me when she introduced "River of Time" on stage by confiding, "There are songs that are hits and there are songs that are heart pieces. This next one is my favorite song my mother has written. It's a message of great loss . . . and then of newly discovered hope."

RIVER OF TIME

I'm holding back a flood of tears
Just thinking 'bout those happy years
Like all the good times that are no more
My love is gone, gone, gone forever more.
Silence so deep only my soul can hear
Says now the past is what I fear
The future isn't what it used to be
Only today is all that's promised me.
Flow on, River of Time,
Wash away the pain and heal my mind.
Flow on, River of Time,
Carry me away

and leave it all far behind.
Flow on River of Time.
We're all driven by the winds of change
Seems like nothing ever stays the same.
It's fate that guides me around the bend
Life's forever beginning, beginning again.
Flow on, River of Time.

My mother-daughter relationship with Wynonna and Ashley will always matter deeply to me. For all of its challenges, I know in my heart that my relationship with my mother will always matter to me, too. There is a new nursing home facility about fifteen miles from my farm. I'm in the process of convincing Mother to allow me move her there, closer to me. I would be able to visit almost daily and she could spend weekends at the farm with us. She would have the chance to spend more time with Wy and her family and Ashley. While it's true that I didn't get my emotional needs met with my mother, I've come to terms with that and now want to give her the best life possible for her remaining years. She is almost ninety years old and very frail, but still displays her quick wit. Surprisingly, she has softened recently and hugs me now and says she loves me. Better late than never. In the long run, she has taught me that no matter what the problem is, compassion is the best answer.

Life is short, but it's wide.

There is no fairy-tale ending to this book, but you and I know there isn't one in real life, either. I still have post-traumatic stress disorder. I'm identifying my triggers so I can avoid them, and I've learned how to process them when they can't be avoided. I very rarely have a panic attack anymore. I also know they won't kill me, that I'll live. I've come to think of them as just occasional nuisances.

I still see and talk to Dr. Rosenbaum in Boston, who monitors my overall condition. I do dialectical behavior therapy with Diana at least once a week and I put into practice the skills I have learned through dialectical behavior therapy, which is my saving grace. I go for sessions in Pilates and I walk my dogs around our farm. I stay occupied with my new heart passions for animals and honoring our veterans. I'm enjoying my friends, again, and have a very active social life. I have my full range of emotions once more.

Larry says, "I've got my wife back!"

Every day I must continue to look forward.

When I had hep C, the reason I survived was hope. Now, once again, I'm living proof of the amazing powers of having a spiritual connection, a support system, humor, a love of nature, goals and a purpose, exercise and nutrition, rest, and an open mind.

During the Judds' Farewell Tour concerts, in every city, every night, I ended with this thought: "I believe in the power of love. And, I believe there is always . . . Hope."

Postscript
Bridge? What Bridge?

A few weeks ago, Larry and I were in Los Angeles, taping an upcoming TV show. As we did every morning, we strolled to a small café in our West Hollywood neighborhood for a cup of coffee. Larry bought a cherry pastry, my favorite, which I envied. We were chatting as I took a bite. I don't know why I bothered, as it had been two and a half years since all food started tasting like paint thinner, an awful and truly rare side effect of the twenty-four electroconvulsive therapy treatments I endured. I had swallowed the mouthful before my eyes flew wide open in surprise. I could taste it. I could taste every sweet, custardy, flakey, delicious bite. My taste buds had miraculously returned.

I've been able to greatly reduce my anti-depression medications to less than half of what they were. My hand still trembles from one that I'm tapering off of, but it should steady out soon.

My hair is still thin and, I'll admit, it's a total hassle to wear a wig or a hat every day, but I know it will grow back in someday, as full, wavy, and red as ever.

Once in a while I'll have a flashback to being locked in a psychiatric ward. I immediately start deep breathing and pull my focus back to the present moment, so I can't think about the past anymore. It's been quite a while since I frantically checked to make sure the doors were unlocked and I could step outside to freedom and fresh air whenever I wanted.

Depression can feel like riding a runaway train. Heart pounding, full speed ahead, with sudden stops, unpredictable curves, frustrating breakdowns, and never knowing what awaits you around the bend.

After the worst three years of my complicated life, I've finally gotten off the train. I've landed on my feet after much hard-won soul-searching, figuring out my troubled past to understand how and why I boarded that horrible train of depression in the first place.

My everyday life is not only manageable, it's even enjoyable once more. I laugh a lot. I'm content and at peace because I practice radical acceptance every single day.

Please join me in telling the truth about depression and anxiety to anyone who will listen. It's a disease of the brain, part heredity, part environment, like heart disease. It's not a character flaw.

Only by telling our stories will more people understand.

Only by telling the truth will we stop the stigma.

I've told my story. Now you know.

And you can tell yours.

You are not alone. I'm still here.

A Note from
Dr. Jerrold Rosenbaum

From the darkest days of her depression, Naomi Judd kept in her view the inspiring thought that she needed to get through all this so she could get a message of hope and help out to others; at the first hints that recovery might be possible, she declared she would write a book about all she has suffered, overcome, learned and experienced to convey a message of understanding and hope and to add another salvo to break down the barrier of stigma. She had emerged from childhood with an extraordinary "double hit" of a genetic pedigree riddled with mental illness and a painful and poignant story of trauma and adversity, but offset remarkably with incredible resilience and determination to endure and overcome. And so we have the gift of her journey shared with us in this authentic, intimate and insightful narrative. I had the privilege of collaborating with her to find a course out of what was an unyielding and severe depression and am moved by her partnership in the shared mission of reducing stigma, increasing hope and finding answers. For all who suffer, there is both compassion and remedy in these pages.

Acknowledgments

M y heartfelt desire is to help others by telling my story and I fully appreciate those who supported my determined goal:

First, love and gratitude to my family: always to my beloved daughters, Ashley and Wynonna, who hold my heart in their hands and always will, and my cherished grandson, Elijah, who lifted my spirits with his dedication to his "Mamaw," along with his sweet Haley. No one carried me through this dark and frightening time more than my husband, Larry. He never left my side and believed in a better day to come, even when I no longer had faith. I am more in love with him now than ever, thirty-seven years strong!

Dr. Mona Lisa Schulz, who has become family to me. Her professional guidance was eclipsed only by her caring and devoted friendship. For more than twenty years she has been a dependable touchstone. Thank you, my friend.

Mel Berger of William Morris Endeavor, thank you for our long association (this is our third book together!) and for your support of this endeavor.

Kate Hartson and her enthusiastic staff at Center Street books, I appreciate your nonstop devotion to this project. The pleasure has been mine.

Marcia Wilkie, thank you for partnering with me on this book. You were a consummate professional on every level and crafted my complicated story in a way that strongly represents the hell I survived and the eventual peace I've found. No easy feat. I feel I've made a new friend.

My management team: Greg Hill and Jeri Cooper and the rest of the staff at Hill Entertainment Group. Thank you for your insightful career guidance and for wrangling new opportunities. Keep 'em coming!

My sincere gratitude to the incredible and gentle mental health professionals who brought me through my toughest trials and held a place for me to find my true self once more: Ted Klontz, PhD, who has been a steady presence for my family for decades; Diana Partington, PhD, who gave me a plan and reminded me that I'm a woman of purpose and passion; and Dr. Jerrold Rosenbaum, who took me on as a patient at my lowest hour and treated my brain disease with dignity. There was great comfort in trusting the exceptional care he provided. Other health care professionals deserving of my appreciation include: Dr. Scott Parker, Dr. W. O'Donnell, Dr. Aaron Milstone, the RNs of the Vanderbilt Psychiatric Unit, and those who have taught me so much: Dr. Francis Collins, Dr. Andrew Weil, Dr. David Perlmutter, and Dr. Dean Ornish.

Many dear friends, both old and new, gave me hope and support. It means so much to me. Thank you: Roy and Helen Snow, Angie Hickman, Sunny Rosenbalm, Casey Martin, Sonya Yontz, Teresa Hughes, Doris McMillan, Doug and Summer Williamson, Don and Christina Potter, Tara Dulin,

Kris Wiatr and staff, Beth Gebhard and staff, the Picnic People, the Ya-Ya's and the Yo-Yo's, and Melanie Shelley, who styled my hair for the book cover.

Finally, to my fellow depression sufferers: I feel such a great fullness in my heart for you, for trusting me with your innermost secrets and vulnerabilities. I have learned as much from you as from the doctors and therapists. Remember, our futures are bigger than our pasts.

MARCIA WILKIE ACKNOWLEDGMENTS

A ton of gratitude to Mel Berger of William Morris Endeavor; working with you is always a true pleasure.

Sincere appreciation to Kate Hartson, executive editor at Center Street; editor Jennifer Josephy; and editorial assistant Grace Tweedy.

A special thank-you to Patricia Bechdolt for her flawless management support.

To Naomi Judd, your story of perseverance and determination has been inspiring. Thank you.

Index